Jill's Best Tips

Smarter ways to burn fat,
stay fit & still enjoy food

JILL BROOK, M.A.

Ten years of painless & practical
willpower-saving strategies.

IBSN 978-0-9830941-2-8

Published by YAMBE Press

at

www.dietforhealth.com

This book is intended solely as a general reference and should not be used as a substitute for medical advice or treatment. Some supplements, fruits and teas may interact with certain medications, so be sure to check with your doctor first before making any changes to your diet. Also, for your safety it is strongly recommended that you get your doctor's approval before beginning any new exercise activities.

Editing, book design, and cover by Melissa Darnell

Table of Contents

A Message from Jill

Eating right, watching your weight, and staying fit is so darn hard! It takes constant vigilance and requires all the willpower you can muster to keep fighting your taste buds, appetite, cravings and an often food-filled environment.

To make the battle a little easier, I'm constantly on the lookout for smart strategies that can either improve success or reduce the effort of the fight.

So for 10 years now I've been sending out practical weekly tips. These are findings from the scientific literature in psychology, nutrition, public health, time management, business, and any other field that has something to offer. Until someone invents the "Magic Pill", these are the best weapons we have. I hope they serve you well!

I'll keep sending weekly tips long after this book is published, so if you'd like to receive them, you can sign up at www.dietforhealth.com.

All my best,

Jill

Giving Thanks Pays Off

Here's a wonderful new research finding: people who take time to appreciate the blessings in their life each day are more motivated to stick with their exercise and healthy eating.

How positive, painless and practical! Why not start now? Take 60 seconds and see how many blessings you can count. Ready, set, begin!

The Laziest Way to Lose Weight

We already knew that sleep deprivation can increase hunger, promote cravings and weaken willpower. But what if you tough it out and don't give in to that urge to splurge?

You can STILL gain weight! A surprising new study compared women who sleep 6 or fewer hours per night to those who sleep 7 or more. Not only did the low-sleepers gain a lot more weight over time, but they were eating less!

It appears as if metabolism, hormones or other factors influenced by sleep can make all the difference to your weight, even if you are eating right.

So now you can feel just as virtuous for going to bed as you do going to the gym!

Feeling Extra Buzzed?

You probably already knew that grapefruit—especially grapefruit juice—can interact with many medications, making them act stronger because it slows the rate at which your liver removes them from your body.

It turns out that grapefruit has the same effect on caffeine. That explains the occasional extra buzz at breakfast!

Caffeine normally has a half-life of about 5 hours, meaning that your body removes half of it in that amount of time. Grapefruit increases the half-life, so you might still be caffeinated at bedtime.

If you are sensitive to caffeine, use this knowledge to fine-tune your intake to avoid jitters and sleepless nights. Sleeping well is essential to health, fitness and weight, so don't let your grapefruit habit mess with it!

Habituation Happens

As my nose grows accustomed to my recently-skunked dogs (ugh!), I am reminded of how all of our senses get desensitized to any stimulus that lasts more than a few moments. In my case, it means I can stand to enter my house again because although the stench is still there, I don't smell it as strongly as I first did. In the case of our taste buds, it means that 90% of the flavor is in the first three bites, and then it quickly fades.

Enjoy and savor those first most-flavorful bites! Then, to fill up, you might as well move on to something VERY healthy.

p.s. Our dog, Lemon, got skunk spray in her mouth, so now her breath is 100% skunk. Thank goodness she probably can't taste it anymore. That is the upside of desensitization!

Healthy Choices that Aren't

Willpower is a limited resource, so I want to make sure you aren't spending any on choices that are less healthy than you think. I see this all the time, and I blame effective advertising for tricking us into believing that some junk food isn't. Here's my list of top offenders:

1) Granola. Read the label, because many kinds are loaded with sugar and oil and the calories can get ridiculous.

2) Graham Crackers. They're mainly sugar and flour.

3) Animal Crackers. Ditto.

4) Cereal Bars. Ditto, but with vitamins and fiber added.

5) Almost All Breakfast Cereal. Read the label and be skeptical of even healthy-looking brands—for example, Heart Smart has more sodium than potato chips.

6) Nutrition Bars. Usually these are candy bars plus vitamins. Read the label.

7) Baked Chips. Baked Lays and many others contain partially hydrogenated fats (i.e. the Grim Reaper Ingredient.)

8) Protein Drinks. Most Americans eat way too much protein, thanks to recent fads. Save your kidneys and feel more satisfied by eating real food with real nutrients.

9) Coffee Mate. OK, you never thought this was healthy, but most people don't realize just how truly unhealthy it is, especially if you use more than one tiny serving per day. Again, it contains partially hydrogenated oils, which contribute to just about every health problem there is.

I'm sure I'm missing some, so please email me the other junk foods that somehow avoided the junky reputation. ...and, if you know how to get such an inflated good reputation, please share because it must be nice!

Vitamin C Helps Fat Burning

A new study found that exercisers deficient in vitamin C burned 25% less fat during an hour on the treadmill. It appears that vitamin C is essential for burning fat because it helps create carnitine, a substance that turns fat into fuel.

So load up on those citrus fruits and green veggies...or risk being robbed of your fat-burning potential!

Feeling Oppressed?

Do you ever feel like eating right means living under a tyrannical regime?! Like maybe there is some sadistic Nutrition Dictator generating lots of complex rules for you to memorize? "Don't eat after 7pm... Avoid white foods... Eat protein with your coffee..." and on and on.

And when he feels ornery, he changes the rules: "Go ahead, eat more eggs!"

The number and complexity of nutrition rules can be overwhelming, so if you want to simplify, here's the only one you need to remember:

When you're hungry, eat how nature intended.

That's it. Every other nutrition truth is just a detail of this main principle, which will take care of your:

- cravings
- weight
- cholesterol
- blood sugar
- heart health
- mood and brain performance

- food addictions
- and just about every other goal, except sports nutrition

My upcoming tips will continue on this theme...so we can all get great results without feeling oppressed by too many rules!

Nature Foods Fight Cravings

Last week I said that eating the way nature intended would address cravings and appetite. Get this:

Research shows that eating foods NOT intended by nature, specifically...

- MSG
- Nutrasweet
- processed sugar, especially high-fructose corn syrup
- high concentrations of salt
- high concentrations of fat
- processed carbohydrates

all can make your brain go crazy for food. They make you want to eat more, eat faster, and make you crave more of those foods later on. Basically, they make you act somewhat addicted, and some people's brains are more susceptible than others'.

When you eat foods intended by nature, your brain doesn't act nearly so addictive. The cravings go away and your appetite becomes less voracious. Your entire body gets more cooperative with your healthy-eating goals.

Sticking with only natural foods isn't always easy, but do the best you can and know that it gets easier with time as your taste buds and appetite quit wanting all the bad stuff.

Viva nature!

Spring Cleaning for Your Body

Continuing with our theme of Nature Foods, here's how they lower cholesterol: it's the soluble fiber.

Any food that is a plant (fruit, veggie, grain, bean, legume, nut or seed) contains indigestible fibers that are like a cleaning crew for your body. The insoluble fibers go through your blood vessels and attach to cholesterol, carrying it out with them when they leave the system, like an efficient janitorial crew for your blood vessels.

Incidentally, there is another kind of plant fiber—insoluble fiber. That's roughage, the janitorial crew for your digestive system. So plant foods scrub out both systems very nicely.

Think of your next salad as "spring cleaning" for your vascular and digestive systems.

Appetizing, eh?

Nature Foods are the Hydration Secret

Here's another way that eating Nature Foods can "kill 2 birds with one snack": they hydrate you, often better than water alone. Here's why:

- Veggies are about 90% water, on average.

- Fresh fruits are about 80% water.

- Whole grains are 60% water.

- Beans, lean proteins and other nature foods are also higher in water than processed or "factory" foods.

...and the water is bound to lots of healthy minerals (i.e. electrolytes) that help your body use the water. What's more, all that water makes you feel full, so you tend to be satisfied on fewer calories.

Here's the exception: if you are exercising in the heat or sweating profusely, you'll want a sports drink. But for everyday normal hydration, water plus fruits and veggies work wonders.

Nature Foods Boost Metabolism

While there are no foods with negative calories (remember the celery myth?), there are indeed foods that burn more calories than others during the digestion process.

Think about what your body does during digestion: it breaks down your food into tiny particles, removes the indigestible fiber (if any), separates out the various nutrients, and then sends them all to the proper place so they can be used or excreted.

Some foods are a lot more work to break down than others, and therefore take more energy (i.e. calories.) Which foods take more energy to break down? You guessed it—Nature Foods.

The reason is fun to visualize. Processed foods were already chopped, mixed and otherwise broken down by the processing plant. The energy that the factory used to break down the food is energy that your body doesn't have to use. For example, when you eat a whole grain, your body needs to break down the food into particles it can absorb and separate the digestible stuff from the fiber. When you eat flour, your body doesn't do that work because the flour mill already chopped the grain into particles and removed the fiber. In a way, flour (or any processed food) is partially "pre-digested". That thought always helps me find processed food less appetizing.

Digesting unprocessed foods is hard work for your body. You can raise your metabolism by up to around 15% by sticking with nature foods. Do the math—that adds up!

Nature Foods are Lower Glycemic

If you haven't heard the term "glycemic index", it refers to how quickly a food boosts your blood sugar. A low glycemic index is preferable to a high one, meaning you want your blood sugar to get a slow and steady rise instead of a quick spike. This is thought to help you lose weight, feel satisfied, avoid cravings and have good energy.

Unprocessed (nature) foods almost always have a lower glycemic index. The explanation is the same as last week's tip about metabolism: Nature Foods take more time and energy to digest. That means the calories are extracted from them more slowly, so they hit your blood stream at a nice, steady, slow rate.

Processed (factory) foods, usually raise your blood sugar more quickly because they digest so quickly— remember, they are "pre-digested" by the processing plant, which did the work of breaking them down, removing fiber, etc.

The more any food has been processed, the more quickly it will be digested and put in your blood stream. The one time you want this is during tough exercise, which is why competitive athletes purposely eat processed foods for quick energy or quick recovery.

So my past half-dozen weekly tips have hopefully convinced you to choose Nature Foods instead of Factory Foods whenever possible. I'll stop beating this dead horse and find a new topic next week.

Cholesterol Tests 101

I often see clients who are disturbed by a high cholesterol test result after years of having healthy results. Often their doctors are insisting they start medication immediately. If this ever happens to you, keep this in mind:

1) Your cholesterol results are highly influenced by what you ate the previous few days. If you normally eat well, but ate junk food the night before your test, it can give you high results. *I see this all the time.* One client had a high result because of a cookie binge on the eve of a blood test, and another client had bad results the day after returning from vacation in Mexico. Both clients had a cholesterol score 100-150 points higher than usual. Two weeks later, after getting back to normal good eating, their scores were back down.

2) The opposite is true. If you kill yourself to eat super-duper-healthy for a week before your test, your cholesterol results will look abnormally good. I don't suggest doing this—you need to know where your cholesterol normally is, not just how good it can get when you eat like a saint.

3) You can buy a home testing kit at the pharmacy for about $20. If you want to experiment with how healthy you need to eat/exercise/etc. to maintain good numbers, you can test as often as you like at home.

4) There are lots of things besides diet that you can do to improve your cholesterol. Come talk to us if you want to try lifestyle changes before medication. I'm happy to say we have a great track record.

Stress Eating Done Right

It goes without saying that it's better to treat stress with laughter, exercise, bubble baths, friends (friends in bubble baths?), etc. than with food. But, let's get realistic.

If you're gonna stress-eat, do it right:

1) Avoid processed foods because they will make you feel worse. Research shows that after the initial, brief mood boost, processed foods actually contribute to depression and anxiety problems. Processed foods are those that came from a factory, not nature.

2) Eat low-glycemic. That way you have time to burn off the extra calories. High-glycemic foods will get stored as fat right away and also make you hungry again sooner.

3) Eat foods with natural mood-boosting properties.

So what should you eat when you are mentally hanging by a thread? Here are my top picks:

1) Pepitas—pumpkin seeds. Raw is healthier, but if you're dying for something crunchy and salty, you can get them roasted and salted. Whole Foods has lots of spiced varieties that are low in salt.

2) Walnuts, almonds, peanuts—in the shell, so you're forced to eat them slowly. Also, busy hands help calm the mind.

3) Nonfat yogurt with flax seeds, cocoa powder and stevia on top. A chocolately mess without the guilt.

Keep in mind that these are not all low-calorie treats, but they are MUCH better than cookies, crackers, and all the other junk you might be contemplating in a moment of stress-induced weakness.

Chew for Success

Chewing your food is even more important than you thought. Get this:

- Chewing more makes you absorb more nutrients from your foods.

- Chewing more helps you eat less because it slows you down.

- New research shows that chewing more makes you stay full longer after you eat.

Big payoff, eh?

So aim for that magic number: 40 chews per bite. That's a lot, but you can do it!

Fattening Food Math

A recent article in the LA Times lamented that calorie and nutrition information listed on products is sometimes incorrect. I find errors all the time, especially on products selling as supposed health food. This is extremely frustrating, but there is only one way to defend yourself: Don't trust any nutrition information that seems too good to be true.

Keep in mind:

1) Especially at restaurants, it is very easy for the chef to add more oil, sugar, etc. than the recipe calls for. It's tempting, too, as this insures great taste.

2) Companies only send a few food items to the Nutrition Lab for calorie and nutrient evaluation. Even Healthy Choice was caught sending different (healthier) versions of their pizza to the Nutrition Lab. The test pizzas had less cheese than the ones you find in stores.

3) By law, a food company can give you MORE quantity than the label states, but not less. For example, I used to buy the Trader Joe's croissants (yes, I indulge) and found they weighed 40% more

than the label stated. That means the calories, fat, etc. are all 40% more also.

Your weight is always a good judge of whether you are eating hidden calories. No matter what the label says, your love handles know the true math.

Human Growth Hormone, the Natural Way

As you probably know (especially if you are a baseball fan), Human Growth Hormone is a hot topic. It's a hormone that is thought to help you stay more muscular, lean, fit and youthful...and it apparently helps you hit grand slams like crazy.

While it is true that your body produces less as you age, there are a number of easy, safe (not to mention, legal) ways to boost HGH production in your body:

- exercise
- adequate sleep
- eating small frequent meals instead of large ones
- avoiding blood sugar spikes and the insulin surge that follows
- losing belly fat

If all that seems like lots of work, think of the baseball players testifying before congress. These things are EASY compared to butt injections and public humiliation, eh?!

Always Hungry?

There's nothing worse than going through the day hungry! If you've got constant hunger, here are some solutions:

1) Are you hungry because you are undereating? If your weight is coming off too fast, we may be underfeeding you! Come on in and we'll find out. In the meantime, fill up on "free foods", like raw veggies, salad with spray dressing, veggie soup and more veggies...

2) Are you sleep-deprived, stressed or exhausted? These things increase appetite, so do your best to manage stress and get a good night's sleep.

3) Drink more water or green tea. Your body easily mistakes thirst for hunger.

4) Chew more. Research shows that you can feel more full on the same amount of food if you chew each bite 40 times. Plus, that will sure slow you down!

5) Try our Bran-a-Crisp crackers or Sprinkles. They are a healthy, high-fiber, super-filling food that you can add to any meal or eat for a snack.

6) Eat red cayenne pepper. This healthy spice has been shown to reduce appetite.

OK, I hope some of these help. If you are currently doing our weight loss program, let us know if you're hungry. Don't suffer in silence!

Truth or Dairy

These days you hear a lot of conflicting advice about whether to eat dairy, so here are some dairy facts to help you decide how much to consume.

Reasons to LOVE dairy:

1) Dairy products are good sources of calcium, potassium, protein and, in the case of yogurt, beneficial probiotics.

2) Dairy is often a super-convenient snack, like low-fat yogurt, string cheese, cottage cheese, etc.

3) A recent study found that people who consume more calcium excrete more dietary fat, rather than absorb it.

4) Another study found that low-fat milk is the best exercise recovery drink. It beat out fancy protein shakes (soy-based or whey-based) for building muscle and burning fat in heavy exercisers.

Reasons to AVOID dairy:

1) You may be lactose-intolerant, in which case you don't digest it. You just become puffy, fluffy or stuffy (inflamed and gassy.) A full 70% of the world lacks the enzymes to fully digest dairy. People of Northern

European descent are most likely to have the right enzymes and people of Asian and African descent are least likely. Of course, you can still do lactose-free dairy.

2) Unless it is organic, many dairy products contain hormones, antibiotics and chemicals used on the farm. These have been blamed for acne and early puberty.

3) Regular (full-fat) dairy is loaded with saturated fat, which is thought to raise cholesterol, contribute to obesity and failure to trigger leptin, the hormone that helps you feel full and satisfied. Fat-free dairy doesn't have this problem.

My advice is to eat organic non-fat dairy if you can digest it well and like it. If you can't eat dairy, you can get your calcium from many other sources, like green veggies, tofu or calcium supplements. And if you don't eat yogurt frequently, you might consider taking another source of probiotics.

More Potassium for Salt Lovers

Here's some good news for folks who love their salt: Increasing potassium helps your blood pressure as much as lowering sodium. Research from Harvard Medical School found that it's the ratio of sodium to potassium—rather than the absolute amount of sodium—that most determines your risk for high blood pressure, stroke and cardiovascular disease.

So, where do you find potassium? In all the healthiest foods: Veggies, fresh fruit, nonfat yogurt, and more veggies, veggies, veggies.

The good news is, now you can justify adding a little salt to those veggies.

Healthy Foods to Get Excited About

When you're adopting better eating habits, it's easy to feel like you've given up everything fun...your favorite sweets, breads, chips, drinks, and everything that makes eating enjoyable! What a bummer!

Eating is undeniably one of life's great pleasures, so we need to keep you excited about healthy foods. Here are my favorite things to get excited about:

- **Tea...**Green tea, red tea, white tea, blue, black and herbal. There are a million different kinds to try, some from exotic places, some that "flower" when you add hot water, some made from interesting herbs and flowers. Try becoming a tea connoisseur...it's healthier AND cheaper than being a wine connoisseur!

- **Spices and herbs...**There are tons of different kinds from all over the world with amazing health properties, like preventing Alzheimer's Disease, improving circulation, boosting metabolism, preventing cancer, reducing joint pain, and lots more. There is a whole world to discover....and you don't need to cook fancy things to use them. I like putting new herb and spice combinations on easy things, like oatmeal, cottage cheese, yogurt, nuts and seeds, chicken breast or anything at all.

- **Exotic fruit...**Go to the section of your grocery store where you pay a little more, but get some intriguing treats, like kumquats, passion fruit, star fruit, boysenberries, and all kinds of nifty unusual things.

- **Seafood...**Go to Fish King or another good seafood supplier and discover how many kinds of seafood you've never tried! Ever eaten octopus? Squid? Unusual shellfish? And don't forget how fun it is to eat ceviche (there are a bunch of different kinds) and crab and lobster straight from the shell.

- **Game meats...**Ostrich, emu and buffalo all have more iron than red meat, with less fat. You can also try lean cuts of elk, rabbit or even guinea pig!

- **Seeds...**Have fun feeling like a hippy by eating hemp seeds, or try chia, golden flax, or the more common pumpkin or sunflower. You can find them all at Whole Foods—just remember to keep the serving size to 1/4 cup.

- **Farmer's markets...**These always help me get re-excited about fresh produce. Be bold and ask the farmers how they enjoy their products. They often have great creative ideas, since they are often eating lots of these foods all season long!

OK, let me know what exciting healthy foods I forgot. Hopefully this helps get you excited about all the tasty treats you can look forward to...without the aftertaste of guilt!

Diet for Happy

Do you ever have a day where your mood isn't good and you aren't sure why? New research suggests that you can blame the crackers...or cookies...or bread...and all processed food.

You already knew that unprocessed food (food that came straight from nature) is better for your health, but new research shows that it's also better for your happiness! One recent study found that people who ate more processed foods were 25% more likely to suffer from depression.

This is interesting to me because many processed foods (especially carbs) can give you a momentary mood lift. This is why we self-medicate with "comfort foods." But in the long term, apparently, they bring us down. So next time you're feeling down, try to have the discipline to forego the quick junk food pick-me-up and invest in your longer-term happiness. Plus, remember that physical activity, laughter, pets and sunlight can give you a quick mood boost without any regret afterwards!

Two New Fat-Fighters

Don't you love it when you can "kill two birds" with one snack? Research shows that two super-healthy foods that we already love can also help prevent weight gain.

1) Turmeric

The yellow spice in curry was already known for being a potent antioxidant and anti-inflammatory, helping to prevent Alzheimer's Disease and other illnesses. New research suggests that it also prevents weight gain, even when you overeat! Granted, the research was done on mice, but when mice were put on a high-calorie, high-fat diet, they stored less fat if they were also eating turmeric.

The best turmeric supplement comes from a company called "NewMark." It's the gold standard because it's organic and unprocessed. You can find it at Whole Foods or my office. You can also just cook with turmeric or sprinkle it on your food.

2) White Tea

You already knew that green tea contains substances that appear to boost metabolism and prevent fat storage. Now researchers are finding that white tea may contain even more of these substances, because it is less processed. The other benefit is that white tea contains even less caffeine (only 10mg/cup) and even more antioxidants.

You can find white tea at most grocery stores or my office. It tastes a lot better than green tea, too!

Put these foods on your grocery list now! You won't find many other habits that give you so much "bang for your buck!"

Willpower for a Healthy New Year!

Happy New Year!

I hope you had a joyous holiday season and enjoyed every tasty morsel that you ate! Now it's time to get your nutrition back on track, so here's a quick review of ways to strengthen your willpower:

1) Get enough sleep (7+ hours for most people).

2) Minimize stress.

3) Prevent low blood sugar by eating small snacks every few hours.

4) Pamper yourself with non-edible treats, like bubble baths, free time, massage, etc.

Research shows that these things make a big difference. Give it a try and remember that the *best* strategy is to minimize your dependence on willpower by getting all leftover holiday treats out of your home ASAP!

Feed on the Facts

Before you bake your favorite holiday treats this holiday season, do yourself a favor: Use the recipe calculator at http://www.caloriecounter.com. It's super easy and quick; simply type in your recipe and it will give you some possibly depressing, but helpful information: The calories, fat, sugar, etc. you are about to consume.

The beauty of this website is that it allows you to change your serving sizes or ingredients, so that when you are horrified by the calories in your holiday cookies, you can retry with different serving sizes or with ingredient substitutions.

If nothing else, this information will help you slow down and savor every bite now that you know the "cost." And, if you'd rather not eat junk this holiday season but still want to fill your home with delicious aromas, try making soups and stews instead of cookies and cakes.

Aggressive Appetite?

This week it seems that everybody has the same question: Why am I so hungry?!

If your appetite has grown recently, here are a few common causes and solutions:

1) The weather. Being cold increases appetite, so bundle up and keep your favorite teas on hand.

2) The holidays. Holiday scents, stress and sleep deprivation can all increase appetite, so make sure to get to bed earlier, schedule some relaxation and throw out any tempting leftovers.

3) TV. Did you watch the football games over Thanksgiving? Next time, use Tivo and skip the ads. Watching TV commercials for snacks and restaurants makes you want to eat more. Interestingly, it also contributes to unrealistic body image issues. What a bummer to want to eat more while simultaneously wanting to be more unrealistically lean and buff!

4) A few "cheats". Did you have a few extra sweet, savory or salty treats for Thanksgiving? Maybe eat 'til you were stuffed? Unless you are a food-saint, probably so! Unfortunately, it only takes a few of these "cheats" to increase your appetite, either because your taste buds were desensitized or because you stretched your stomach. If this is the case, you'll have to ride this one out and wait for your body to return to its normal state. It's worth it—you don't want to keep your stomach in its post-Thanksgiving stretched state.

Two other solutions are peppermint tea and red cayenne pepper. They've both been shown to reduce appetite.

If that doesn't work, just stick your tongue to a frozen pole. Just kidding! Anyone who has ever done this, as I have, knows it isn't nearly as funny as it sounds...

Sugar Suppresses Immunity

As you do your best to avoid catching a cold or flu this winter, keep this in mind: For 30 minutes to 5 hours after eating sugar, your immune system is weakened and you are more likely to get ill. In fact, one study found that 100g of sugar (equivalent to 2 sodas) reduced the ability of white blood cells to kill germs by 40%.

This means that you need to avoid sugar at these times:

- at the first sign of a cough or sniffles
- when exposed to sick people
- when at school, on a plane, or in a crowded area
- whenever you want your immune system at it's best.

Gosh—you might as well give up eating sugar all together!

Great idea.

Healthier Holiday Fun

It is said that the average American gains 8 pounds over the holidays. Yikes! Here's our Top 10 list of holiday traditions and treats that are healthier AND more fun than pigging out. Plan NOW to include them this year!

10) Fill a pinata with toys, stickers and coins and let your kids go at it. (I don't have kids, so I fill it with dog toys and let the dogs tear it apart).

9) Make holiday soups and stews instead of cookies.

8) String cranberries and popped corn to make lovely (and tasty) garland.

7) Go for a holiday hike, picnic or mini-golf game.

6) Find a fun or funny game to play during cocktail hour...one that makes it hard to eat and drink too much. Card games keep your hands busy (making it harder to eat) and you sure can't beat Twister!

5) Instead of making a gingerbread house (which has way too many temptations), consider making a

different, non-edible craft, like a wreath or ornament.

4) Get in the spirit by sampling holiday teas and coffee blends. I'm told that Peet's Holiday Blend coffee is outstanding.

3) Want a holiday baking challenge without the sugar? Try making Turducken. That's a chicken inside a duck inside a turkey and only a brave few have ever made it.

2) Round up all the tempting packaged food in your kitchen and donate it to a food bank for the holidays.

1) Ask for healthy holiday gifts, like spa treatments, fitness gear, gym memberships, personal training sessions, kitchen appliances and other presents that will get you healthier for the new year.

What have I missed? Please send me your ideas!

Why Every Bite Matters

As we enter the holiday season, it gets SO VERY EASY to let down your guard and eat more junky foods, even if it's just a bite here and there. Here are 4 reasons to stay vigilant:

1) One indulgence (with sweets, for example) can start "taste bud ping pong", where you then crave salt, which makes you crave more sweets... and on and on. Research show that your brain fails to send satiety signals in this situation, so it is extremely hard to stop eating.

2) Even small quantities of over-flavored food (e.g. super salty, sweet, rich, etc.) can desensitize your taste buds so that your next healthy meal tastes bland and unsatisfying. Ever eaten an apple after a cookie? It tastes like nothing.

3) A single bad meal can raise your risk of heart attack and stroke for 5-12 hours, as the unhealthy fats course through (and potentially clog) your cardiovascular system. On the up-side, a single healthy meal can lower your risk. In fact, you can

lower your cholesterol, blood pressure, blood sugar and triglycerides with a single day of eating right. Don't believe me? Get a home cholesterol/blood sugar/blood pressure kit at the pharmacy and see for yourself. It's quite motivating!

4) Every new eating habit begins with a single decision and is strengthened or weakened by each subsequent bite that you take. That means every bite DOES matter, because habits are the key to lifelong success. With every good choice, the next one gets easier to make.

Now that I've ruined your enjoyment of holiday sweet treats, next week I'll send some ideas for healthy, tasty, fun alternatives. I don't want you thinking I'm the Grinch, after all.

Peter Piper's Appetite Suppressor

Some new research suggests that red cayenne pepper helps keep you feeling full longer. One study found that folks ate fewer calories all day—without realizing it—when they added this spice to their foods. If you are watching your weight, try adding it to:

- eggs and omelets
- chicken, fish, turkey, protein dishes
- soups and stews
- salads
- veggies
- salsas
- hot cocoa
- or anything else

Let me know if it works for you!

Kill 3 Birds with 1 Onion

With school back in session, cold and flu germs travel faster than ever! Remember that you can protect yourself by eating foods rich in quercitin, like:

- apples
- blueberries
- broccoli
- spinach
- lettuce
- onions
- or best of all...red onions

They have 4 times the quercitin of the other foods. Raw or cooked is great, although the quercitin may be better absorbed if the food is cooked. Quercitin is an antioxidant, which means that it will also help protect you from pollution and premature aging.

Try slowly cooking red onions until they are soft and sweet. They make great flavorings for chicken, salads, fish or all by themselves.

Stop Wine-ing

One of the happiest bits of nutrition research to date has always been that moderate drinking prevents heart attacks. It was thought to be good for your heart in many of the same ways that exercise is good for your heart—by lowering blood pressure, reducing stress, decreasing inflammation, etc.

A recent study in the American Journal of Health Promotion found that moderate drinkers exercise more than non-drinkers, so THAT may be the reason for the connection between alcohol and heart health. Doh!

More research will uncover the truth, but remember that alcohol—whether good or bad for your heart—is always bad for weight loss. It increases your appetite, suppresses your metabolism, interferes with muscle recovery and about half of the calories turn directly to fat.

Besides, there are a bunch of weight-friendly things you can do for your heart: Laugh, volunteer, get a dog, meditate, do yoga, sleep more, drink tea and, of course, eat your fruits and veggies.

Sorry for the bad news!

Fabulous Forgotten Food Group

What if there was a category of foods that tasted amazing, had almost no calories and had health properties that put veggies to shame? Good news...there is!

It's herbs and spices. If you've gotten away from using these at every meal, you're missing out. Not only do they allow you to get flavor without salt, sugar and fat, but they also do great things for your health, like:

- Cinnamon helps reduce blood sugar and cholesterol and can help calm your stomach.

- Cayenne and red pepper flakes contain compounds that prevent cancer.

- Ginger has loads of benefits—it's an anti-inflammatory, circulatory stimulant and digestive aid. Being an anti-inflammatory means that it helps your health in a bunch of ways, including possibly preventing Alzheimer's, heart disease, arthritis and more.

- Parsley and basil are full of antioxidants and so many different nutrients that you should always eat the sprig that comes to adorn your plate.

- Turmeric is the yellow spice in Indian food and appears to be the reason that Alzheimer's Disease is rare there. It is a potent anti-inflammatory and antioxidant, which means it helps you live longer and better in a bunch of different ways. Research keeps connecting inflammation to more diseases, including inflammatory bowel, arthritis, autoimmune problems, heart disease and more.

I could go on and on about other herbs and spices, but you get the idea: They are all very potent little morsels of flavor and health!

Use them often—every chance you get—and splurge on ones that are fresh and of high quality. Hey, when you're giving up so many other sources of flavor (i.e. sugar, salt, fats, chemicals) you deserve it!

p.s. YOU DON'T HAVE TO BE A GREAT COOK! Add cinnamon, cloves, allspice, etc. to your cereal or fruit or yogurt, Add dill, rosemary, cayenne pepper, etc. to your cottage cheese. Drink ginger tea or chai tea, which has a lot of spices. You don't have to cook to fit herbs and spices into your life.

Flames Need Flavenoids

With the wildfires currently raging on, I hope this finds you safe. Once you have protected your family and your irreplaceable belongings, it is time to consider your lungs. The air quality is terrible, but there are some substances in food that help protect you from lung damage: flavenoids.

Flavenoids are the pigments in fruits, veggies, and any plant food. Flavenoids serve as anti-inflammatory aides, and they prevent DNA damage to your cells. Make sure to get some of these throughout the day so that you will always have some "lung defenders" coursing through your body. All fruits, veggies and teas have them, but here are the very best sources for lung protection:

- apples (especially red)
- strawberries
- tea—green or black, decaf or regular
- onions

- beans
- broccoli
- brussels sprouts

And if you are a smoker, you need to eat loads of these foods for the rest of your life.

I know many of you have homes that are in danger. I'm sending you all my best wishes!

Surviving Summer Slump

In the past 10 years that I've been doing nutrition counseling, I've noticed something that I can't explain: I call it the Summer Slump and we're in the thick of it.

What is Summer Slump? It's a week or two where almost everyone struggles with motivation, mood and/or willpower. Of course, it's common for everyone to have times when they struggle with these things, but for some reason almost EVERYONE is struggling right now.

Why? I don't know! Maybe it's the heat, end of summer vacation, or alignment of the planets. If you have a guess, please let me know. At any rate, here's what to do about it:

1) Make sleep a priority. It will reduce appetite and cravings and improve energy and willpower.

2) Splurge on yummy summer produce. If over-eating peaches will keep you from over-eating cookies, it's well worth it!

3) Realize that these doldrums are normal and will pass. In the meantime, try not to do anything you regret too much.

4) Keep fighting your best fight! At every single meal, make the best choices that you can. Whatever the situation and whatever your willpower, DO YOUR BEST with it. Even if that means eating 6 scoops of ice cream instead of 8, it still makes a difference. Never give up. 90% of the damage happens only after you say "scr*w it."

5) Come on in and see us at DfH. When you least feel like it is probably when you most need to!

Summer Produce and Pesticides

If you are wondering when it's worth it to pay more for organics, here's the "dirt" on how to prioritize.

Types of produce MOST likely to contain pesticide residue (i.e. try to get organic):

- peaches
- apples
- sweet bell peppers
- celery
- nectarines
- strawberries
- cherries
- pears
- grapes (imported)
- spinach
- lettuce

- potatoes

Types of produce LEAST likely to contain pesticide residue (i.e. organic not a priority):

- papayas
- broccoli
- cabbage
- kiwis
- bananas
- sweet peas (frozen)
- asparagus
- mangoes
- pineapple
- sweet corn (frozen)
- avocados
- onions

No matter whether you can afford/find organic or not, remember it is ALWAYS a good choice to eat more produce. Most health and weight problems in America can be prevented by eating more produce and less processed food, NOT by avoiding produce out of worries about chemicals.

p.s. The lists above came from the Environmental Working Group, a nonprofit organization.

Go on the Offensive

This morning's news included a story about a lawsuit aiming to get cancer warnings on hot dog packages. It's true that processed meats increase the risk of colon cancer. That got me thinking about how a *bazillion* things—many unavoidable—also appear to increase cancer risk, including...

- undercooked foods
- overcooked (charred) foods
- heated starches
- too much folic acid (added to foods, like bread, to prevent neural tube defects)
- not enough soy
- too much soy
- inhaling near a car, leaf-blower or any vehicle
- living in a city (smog)
- living in the country (farm chemicals)
- too much sunlight
- not enough sunlight (vitamin D deficiency)

- not enough intercourse (for men...prostate cancer)
- X-rays
- cell phones, maybe
- flying at high altitudes (atmospheric radiation)
- parking in underground structures
- common ingredients in soaps, lotions and cosmetics
- sleep deprivation
- stress
- NOT bearing children (although *having* them pretty much guarantees more sleep deprivation!)
- plastic food containers
- bottled water
- NOT undereating
- and, most of all, *aging*!

OK, you get the picture. Almost everything! Life itself is cancer-inducing!! You can't possibly avoid every risk! Oh nooooo! What should you do?

For one thing, you can GET PROTECTED FROM THE INSIDE: eat an anti-cancer food every few hours and you'll be giving your body what it needs to defend itself as best it can. What foods protect you?

PLANTS! Veggies, fruits, whole grains, nuts, seeds, legumes, beans, herbs, spices and teas. Work these foods into every meal and snack and your blood will be coursing with an army of protectors.

And, as luck would have it, those are the same foods that protect you from heart disease, diabetes, high blood sugar, obesity and premature aging. It's almost like the "magic pill" has existed all along....in nature.

So get some of these foods at EVERY MEAL and let me know if you manage to live forever.

p.s. I didn't mean to scare anyone with that long list of cancer-causers. Keep in mind that DRIVING is a bigger health risk than all those things put together!

Coffee Lovers Rejoice

Good news! You can officially stop feeling guilty about your coffee habit:

Two new studies suggest that coffee can prevent, and maybe even somewhat reverse, Alzheimer's Disease. What's more, many studies show that caffeine can improve mood, alertness and energy, help prevent diabetes, Parkinson's disease, and liver cancer, decrease the risk of stroke and may help prevent skin cancer and eye damage from the sun. It also increases endurance in athletes.

But BEFORE you rush out to buy a latte and stock in Starbucks, here are some warnings about increasing your caffeine intake too quickly:

1) Watch out for insomnia, edginess, the jitters, diarrhea, etc.

2) It will act as a diuretic for the first few weeks until your body adjusts to it, so watch out for dehydration and eat extra minerals like calcium to replace what you lose.

3) Keep in mind you'll become dependent—you will probably have headaches if/when you don't have your normal amount.

4) It will probably raise your blood pressure for the first few weeks also, so if you have blood pressure issues, check with your doctor first.

Kumquat with Me...

Hopefully you will go grocery shopping today to stock up on convenient, healthy foods for the week. For something novel, try kumquats.

This year's crop of kumquats is amazing—sour on the inside with sweet skins (yes, you eat the skin). Willie Wonka himself couldn't have created a funkier taste experience. PLUS they are nature's perfect convenience food—keep 'em in your pocket all day long and pop one in your mouth whenever you get hungry. 8 of them counts as 1 serving of fruit. Enjoy!

Eat for 3 Hours and Lose Weight?!

Here's an interesting finding:

In France, the average person spends over 2.5 hours per day eating and drinking.

In America, the average person spends about 0.6 hours per day eating and drinking, yet is more overweight.

No fair! What gives?!

It turns out that the French just eat slower and manage to eat FEWER calories, despite spending so much MORE time eating.

How's that for simple? We just need to SLOW DOWN! Chew more, set down your fork, eat left-handed, do whatever it takes to make the pleasant experience of eating last a little longer.

Bon Appetite!

A Reason to Buy the Cow

As you may know, I'm not a fan of post-workout shakes and drinks unless you work out very intensely and can't get enough calories from food...a rare problem! But new research shows that even if you would benefit from a protein drink, there's a surprising best choice: milk.

Yes, plain old boring nonfat milk.

In a recent study, bodybuilders drank either nonfat milk or one of several protein shakes right after their heavy workouts. Every few weeks, body fat and muscle were measured.

Surprisingly, the nonfat milk beat out all of the fancy schmancy protein drinks—both soy-based drinks and whey-based. Milk was the best in terms of both fat loss AND muscle gain!

This is just one more finding that shows Mother Nature serves us better than our own man-made creations. So quit wasting money on fancy protein drinks, unless you are lactose-intolerant AND can't get enough post-workout calories from food. In that case, a soy protein-based drink may be right for you.

Scary Supplements

You may have heard that the best-selling weight loss supplement, Hydroxycut, was recently recalled because of reports of liver damage, heart damage and other problems. At least one user even died from it. This reminds us that there is, so far, no magic pill. Anything that seems too good to be true...you know the rest.

Next time you are considering buying dietary supplements of any kind, beware. Two recent studies by independent laboratories found that fewer than half of supplements contain the ingredients listed in the promised amounts. They also found that some supplements were contaminated with lead or other pollutants.

There are some very healthy and beneficial supplements out there, but there are many more questionable ones. I only trust supplements that have been third-party tested by groups without a profit motive, like a well-respected university. Only a handful of supplement companies do that, and it will cost you more, but you probably don't want to put anything in your body that hasn't been freely and honestly tested.

When the magic pill arrives, don't worry—I'll tell you! ...and then we'll joyfully eat chocolate chip cookies the rest of the day...

The Secret to Self-Control

Ever wonder why some people are able to resist tasty temptations better than others? Is it pure discipline? Strength of will? Genetics? Maybe partially, but get this:

Self control is largely the ability to self-distract.

Research from Stanford suggests that a person's ability to refrain from eating something tasty largely depends on whether they are able to distract themselves with a different activity.

Whoa! Think about that for a minute. Could it really be that simple?

Apparently! In their studies, they had youngsters sit in a room with a tempting treat (a marshmallow). The kids were told that if they could resist the marshmallow, they would get MORE treats later on. About 1/3 of the kids were able to resist the temptation, and it was almost always because they would do things to distract themselves—sing, jump around, use the marshmallow as a toy car, etc. Those kids that just sat there almost always caved in. Interestingly, the kids who could distract themselves in the face of temptation also went on to have higher grades, better jobs, better health and other rewards that require delaying gratification.

If you struggle with eating bad foods or eating too much, then give this a try: instead of focusing on NOT eating, focus on DOING something else...anything else!

And if you want to read a much more detailed article, see "Don't! The Secret of Self-Control" in the May 18th, 2009 New Yorker Magazine.

Don't Drink Your Calories

One of the EASIEST ways to lose weight is to stop drinking any of your calories. Many studies show that solid food calories register with your appetite, so you naturally eat less at your next meal without even trying. Liquid calories don't.

On average, studies show that consuming 100 extra calories...

- in solid form, leads folks to eat 65 fewer calories at their next meal
- in semi-solid form, leads to 21 fewer calories
- in liquid form, leads to eating NO fewer calories

The reason is ghrelin, the hormone that makes you want to eat. Ghrelin levels go down—and stay down—longer after solid food.

You Bet!

Here's a fun finding: a recent study found that people got better weight loss results when they made a monetary bet with someone about it.

The thinking is that when your willpower is weak, your pride or thrift may still save you from eating poorly. It may also give you a fun challenge (instead of a grueling one) and more social support. Try this for any habit you want to change.

Have fun with it and let me know if it works for you!

More Gain from Your Pain

If you make the time to exercise, here are 5 ways to get more bang for your buck:

1) Enjoy your coffee or tea before your workout and not after. Caffeine helps you access fat, decreases muscle pain and helps you exercise harder longer. Don't drink it afterwards or on rest days because the more caffeine you consume, the more you habituate to the effect.

2) Drink green tea right before or during your workout. I suggest icing it and putting it in your sports bottle. Research suggests that green tea increases your metabolic afterburn, so it keeps you burning extra calories after a workout.

3) Eat within 1 hour of finishing a killer workout. Your muscle cells will soak up the carbs and protein you eat so that they recover faster and stronger for next time.

4) Include intense intervals. A few intense intervals will make you burn more fat the entire workout and

will extend your metabolic afterburn. Intensity also increases longevity and makes your cells act younger, by increasing the amount of oxygen they can consume.

5) Avoid alcohol for 24 hours after a killer workout. It interferes with recovery. The whole reason you worked out hard was to break down muscle so that it would grow back stronger and better! Don't do a hard workout if you don't plan to allow yourself adequate recovery.

Happy sweating!

Winning the Sugar War

The average American eats over 20 teaspoons of added sugar every day. Yikes! Everybody **knows** they should avoid processed sugar, but **knowing** isn't all that helpful...***Doing*** it is the hard part! Here is what the latest research says about winning your war against sugar:

- Watch out for taste bud ping pong. When a sweet flavor is eaten along with a salty one—think French fries with soda or pretzels with juice—the brain doesn't get satiated and it is very difficult to stop eating.

- Push the fruit after exercise. Fruit (which is about 80% water) tends to taste better after exercise because a thirsty body prefers watery foods.

- Sweeten it yourself. Buy breakfast cereals, drinks, and other snacks with NO sugar and then add your own, if you need to sweeten it. This makes you much more aware of how much sugar you consume.

- Serve protein at each meal. This helps keep blood sugar levels steady, which can help prevent cravings.

- Make sleep a priority. Sleep deprivation can lead to sugar cravings.

- Finally, avoid even the occasional sugar binge. Why? Psychology researchers at Princeton have finally proven that sugar is addictive. Granted, they studied rats (so they could look inside their brains), but they found that eating sugar produces results similar to taking addictive drugs. Rats fed sugar had altered brain chemistry similar to drug addicts; they had cravings, withdrawal, relapse and even increased preference for alcohol. Perhaps reclassifying sugar as an addictive substance will help us have the discipline not to buy it or keep it in the house.

Fight a good fight for me!

Stress Solution, Part 1

As you may have experienced, stress makes it harder to lose weight—not only because it can affect your appetite and willpower, but also because it can raise your blood sugar. How? Adrenaline.

Adrenaline helps prepare your body for the Fight-or-Flight Response (i.e. exercise), which includes raising your blood sugar. High blood sugar is great if you need to outrun a predator, but bad if you want your fat cells to open up and let out some energy to burn. You body doesn't know whether your stress comes from your job or a hungry tiger chasing you, so it errs on the side of survival.

What can you do about it?

1) **Exercise more when you are stressed:** Give your body the physical activity it prepared for. You'll be surprised how energized you are with the help of your adrenaline.

2) **Eat fewer carbohydrates.** When your adrenaline is already raising your blood sugar, you can

compensate by eating foods that don't raise your blood sugar as much, like proteins, veggies and a little healthy fat, like nuts or olive oil. You don't need to eat carbs when your blood sugar is already high from adrenaline.

Hope you don't need this week's tip.

Stress Solutions, Part 2

Last week I told you that when stress is higher, your carb intake should be lower (bummer, I know!). So here's some good news about what you should eat *more* of when stress abounds:

Foods rich in the calming nutrients magnesium and omega-3 fatty acids.

Magnesium-rich foods include...

- cocoa powder (sprinkle it on fruit, cottage cheese, oatmeal, etc. with a little stevia or your favorite sweetener)
- halibut
- white beans
- wheat bran
- spinach

Omega-3-rich foods include...

- cold-water fatty fish like wild salmon, trout, haddock, mackerel, sardines

- fish oil supplements
- flax seed oil
- walnuts (limit to 1/4 cup per serving)

If you want the most omega 3's for the least calories, fish oil supplements are your best bet. Look for a brand that says "3rd party certified" to make sure they don't contain mercury. Some studies have shown that fish oil has such a powerful effect on mood and anxiety that some folks on antidepressant or anti-anxiety medication have been able to lower their doses after starting fish oil supplements. Wow!

Cheap Tricks

The terrible economy has got me thinking about new ways to be healthier, and I've been thrilled to find there are some cost-cutting measures that are great for your health and waistline. Here are my favorites:

1) Buy smaller apples, potatoes, zucchini, eggplant or any produce with an edible skin. The skin is the healthiest part of the food, and smaller items have a higher ratio of skin to insides (remember your middle school geometry?). That means it's better to eat 2 small apples than 1 big one. The smaller produce is usually cheaper, so shhhh...don't tell the grocers that it's superior.

2) Eat more beans and lentils. For the cost of one pound of chicken breast from Whole Foods, you could eat lentils for a week! Just make sure to count them as your protein AND your starch, since they are rich in both. Serve them with lots of veggies, since they aren't quite as filling (per calorie) as animal protein.

As if the cost weren't reason enough, new research is showing that replacing animal protein with plant protein lengthens your life. That means making a big pot of lentils or beans once a week with lots of garlic, ginger, herbs or spices is your personal and super-convenient fountain of youth!

3) Drink tap water instead of bottled. It is at least as healthy.

4) Replace cold boxed cereals (expensive and highly processed) with whole grains like oats, brown rice, bulgar or any other boiled whole grain. Just compare—for the cost of 8 servings of Cheerios you get 60 servings of oatmeal!

5) And, of course, a few no-brainers: eat out less, drink water instead of other beverages, and eat more slowly so that you are less likely to overeat.

Daylight Savings, Stay Light, Cravings

Daylight Savings Time is early this year and that is good news for your diet:

1) Our body chemistry is better at storing fat later in the day, which is why it's better to eat bigger breakfasts and smaller dinners. Daylight Savings Time helps because staying awake longer and being more active after dinner helps prevent the post-dinner blood sugar rise that causes weight gain. **Best bet: eat early and get out for a walk after dinner.**

2) Appetite and cravings increase after dark. That's why we tend to crave pizza, not veggies, at 11pm. **Best bet: Minimize these dangerous dark hours by going to bed early.**

3) Being cold makes you hungrier. Hooray for warmer weather!

So take advantage of the longer days and make me proud! :)

Crash and Burn with Eating Auto-Pilot

The average football fan consumes an estimated 1200 calories while watching the Super Bowl, and the numbers are similar for movie-watchers. Watching anything while eating tends to put viewers on "eating auto-pilot", and the worst part is that they probably don't even taste most of those calories. Here's why: Habituation.

After the first bite of any food, your taste buds start to desensitize. That means they get used to the flavor and stop noticing it as much. By the 10th bite, you barely taste anything at all. All of your senses— touch, smell, hearing, sight, taste—do this in response to any repeated stimulus. It's just like when your eyes adjust to bright light or you put on perfume and don't notice it after 20 seconds.

This means that 90% of the pleasure of any decadent food comes in the first few bites. Savor and enjoy those bites then either quit eating or fill up on something healthy. Don't swallow any junk you aren't going to fully taste!

Sordid Sweets and Salts

With Super Bowl snacks soon upon us, it's time to remind you that you shouldn't mix your salty and sweet snacks. Why? Get this:

When you eat only 1 flavor at a time, your brain gets quickly satisfied, which means you choose to stop eating before too long. When you eat 2 or more complimentary flavors together (sweet and salty, bitter and sweet), your brain *never gets tired* of eating! One flavor enhances the experience of the other and your brain is so happily over-stimulated that you won't want to stop eating until you are ready to burst!

Food producers and sellers know this and use this to boost sales. Ever wonder why all coffee houses sell sweets or why there are free salted peanuts at bars? Food companies even hide lots of unnecessary salt in sweet cereals, just to make your brain demand more. This all means that you can reduce your appetite and reach satiety sooner if you stick to one flavor at a time.

Make sure to watch out for beverage flavors too because even diet drinks, if sweet, will keep you from ever getting tired of a salty or savory meal.

And remember that it is extra good karma for your team if you have veggies and low-fat dip as your Super Bowl snack!

Pressure Pointers

Many of us consider salt a nearly-free food. It has no calories and after we've sworn off sugar, flour and fat we think we deserve *some* flavor, right?

It turns out that excess salt is quite a killer. Just to get our attention, the Center for Science in the Public Interest has publicized these frightening factoids:

- 90% of Americans have high blood pressure by the time they reach 70.

- High blood pressure kills Americans at the rate of a 747 crashing daily.

Whoa! You don't want to be on that flight, so here's what you can do: in addition to cutting sodium to under 1500mg/day: increase potassium. The ratio of these two minerals determines your blood pressure. Most Americans eat too little potassium, which compounds the sodium problem. Here's the good news: foods you should be eating anyway—fruits, veggies, low-fat dairy—are chock-full of potassium. It won't hurt to relax, lose weight and work up a good sweat several times per week, either.

Resolution Solution

Happy New Year!

By now you've chosen your New Year's Resolutions, so here's how to maximize your chances of sticking to them!

The most important thing is to make your resolutions very **specific, realistic and measurable** on a daily basis. For example, "losing 10 pounds by April" is too general and it's difficult to know if you've done your part every day. Try breaking that goal into specific behaviors that will help you accomplish it. Examples of good resolutions are:

- Eat a breakfast that contains some protein every morning.

- Eat a salad, with dressing on the side, once per day.

- Don't allow any junk food in the cupboards.

- Keep an honest food journal.

These are good resolutions because they aren't too difficult and don't leave any room for fudging. Yet, when you do them every day, they add up to lots of results. So think about how you could break down your resolutions—whatever they are—into specific, realistic, measurable behaviors. Do it **_right now_** and see how it motivates you to accomplish your goals each day.

Tips for New Exercisers

Hello Bootcampers (and all others starting a tough workout program)!

By now you are probably tired, sore, sleep-deprived and wondering why you haven't lost any weight yet (answer: fluid retained in swollen muscles). This may be the moment you are considering rewarding yourself with a tiny tasty cheat-treat...just a small one...nothing too terrible...maybe just a bite?

The latest research shows at least 5 reasons to tough it out and avoid having even a single cheat bite. Staying on track 100% is worth it because:

1) It will instill habits faster. Healthy behaviors become automatic after a while, and that's when you've got it made because they no longer require willpower. It takes less than half the time to cement in habits when you start by sticking to them 100%. It's like training your dog. Ever made the mistake of allowing your dog to break the rules just once? It buys you weeks of extra work! Your brain is sadly similar to your pooch.

2) It changes your taste buds. A single bite of something that is unnaturally sweet, salty or savory will over-stimulate your taste buds and desensitize them for days or weeks. Now everything else you eat tastes more bland. Staying away from junky food allows your taste buds to re-sensitize and get more enjoyment from every bite. It usually takes 1-2 weeks, and boy is it great when veggies and other formerly-boring foods start to have complex and delightful flavors.

3) It reduces your appetite. A single splurge can send your blood sugar soaring, which leads to increased appetite later on. It becomes a vicious cycle.

4) It reduces cravings. For the same reason as above: blood sugar.

5) It frees your mind. Exciting new research is showing that the old advice to enjoy your treats "in moderation" is for the birds! Occasional treats just keep you excited for the next one. When people just give up something permanently, they are more likely to forget about it and never miss it.

I know how hard you are working and how much you deserve a treat—so make it a non-edible one, like a bubble bath or massage. In later weeks I'll share tips for "cheating" and getting away with it, but for now, being 100% on track will make it easier to get great results and maintain them for life. So re-read your nutrition guide and keep this message handy for any moments of weakness. Your future super-fit self will thank you.

Make me proud!

Tuna Tips

You've probably heard the bad news...the healthiest, most convenient, low-calorie protein around, canned/bagged tuna, may contain high levels of mercury. Well, here are 2 bits of good news:

1) You can now get skinless, boneless **salmon** in a packet or can, which looks and tastes almost like tuna.

2) If you buy "chunk light" instead of "albacore" canned tuna, it typically has only 25% as much mercury and also has less fat.

Sweat the Small Stuff

Well, the latest numbers are in and Americans are now gaining 2 pounds per year, every year, on average. That's 20 pounds per decade—yikes!

Consider this: to gain 2 pounds per year you need to overeat by only 19 calories per day (1 saltine cracker). On the bright side, this also means that you can lose 2 pounds per year by burning 19 calories more than you eat each day—that's only 2 extra minutes of exercise. Every little nibble or extra minute of physical activity adds up over time, so start sweating the small stuff.

Sugar is Finally Proven Addictive

Psychology researchers at Princeton have finally proven what you may have already suspected. Granted, they studied rats (so they could look inside their brains), but they found that eating sugar produces results similar to taking addictive drugs. After allowing rats to binge on sugar, they found:

1) Altered brain chemistry: The rats' dopamine receptors were fried, just like with drug addicts.

2) Cravings: The rats went through withdrawal when their sugar was taken away.

3) Relapse: The rats ate even larger amounts of sugar at their next opportunity.

4) Alcoholism: The rats started drinking much more alcohol after becoming addicted to sugar.

Perhaps re-classifying sugar as an addictive substance will help us have the discipline not to buy it or keep it in the house.

Now perhaps those Princeton researchers can get to work on finding us something pleasurable that isn't illegal, immoral or fattening!

Winter Weight Woes

If you've noticed that it's harder to watch your weight lately, you're not crazy. Winter weather and shorter days are tough on willpower and fat-burning for a few reasons:

1) Being cold increases your appetite.

2) Cravings for comfort food increase after the sun sets and it's dark outside.

3) Exercising in colder weather doesn't work your heart as hard. When your heart has to pump enough blood to simultaneously fuel you **and** cool you (i.e. sweat), you burn more calories.

4) It's good TV season. Who can be bothered to be active after dinner when a new episode of your favorite show is on?!

What should you do?

Fight your best fight until the weather gets warmer and be glad you live in Southern California! Think of all those poor folks who live up north and live like this until almost June!

Your Body's Sugar "Storage Tanks"

New research has found that some people are prone to releasing more insulin than others after eating carbohydrates. Insulin moves carbohydrates out of your blood stream and into storage—which is usually your fat cells—so these high-insulin-releasers are more likely to gain weight unless they maintain a low-carb diet.

This explains why some lucky folks get away with eating more carbs than others.

If you believe you might be one of those unlucky carb-sensitive weight-gainers (or if you just love your carbs and want to avoid storing fat after eating them), here's a solution:

Build bigger muscles and use them regularly.

Before storing fat, your body will store sugar in your muscles as glycogen...but only if there is space for it. When you exercise your muscles, you burn up some of the muscle sugar, making room for more. Think of muscles as your sugar "storage tanks" that give you freedom to enjoy more carbs.

Now you know why I lift weights!

Taste Buds Gone Wild—The MSG Story

Yesterday I gobbled down an entire bag of white cheddar rice cakes. They were so delicious I couldn't stop. I was in a trance of pleasure and I was helpless! And after I polished off the bag and wished for more, it dawned on me that there must be some MSG hiding in there. That's the salty additive that makes sane folks eat like the world is ending.

But the label didn't list MSG. Instead the label said "yeast extract", which is code-word for MSG. How tricky!

So here's a quick primer on MSG:

1) MSG is considered an "excitotoxin," which means that it makes food taste *amazing*. Your brain's pleasure center goes wild upon tasting it and your appetite balloons.

2) People eat more quickly and much more food when their meals are laced with MSG.

3) A Chinese study looked into why MSG-eaters were more likely to be overweight and obese. The

simple explanation was that they were eating a whole lot more.

4) MSG is often hard to identify on a label—it sneaks into things like:

- yeast extract
- hydrolyzed vegetable protein
- sodium and calcium caseinate
- autolyzed yeast
- hydrolyzed corn protein
- texturized vegetable protein

It is also sometimes sprayed on commercial crops to stimulate growth.

5) There is some evidence that MSG can cause chronic overproduction of insulin and can also damage the hypothalamus, which controls hunger. The many claims about cancer don't have strong support.

Chances are that you will have a tough time identifying MSG, especially when eating out. My suggestion is to pay attention to which foods drive your taste buds unnaturally wild and then assume the worst.

If you already struggle with overeating, MSG is probably a disaster for you. Do your best to avoid it and seek out some healthy herbs and spices instead. At least now you can lose the guilt: your lack of control isn't you. It's the MSG.

Law and Order and Weight Gain

You probably already knew that watching TV increases hunger (thanks to commercials) and contributes to body image problems (thanks to stars' perfect bodies), but here's a doozie: *watching TV suppresses your metabolism below its basal rate!*

Researchers recently measured the calorie burn associated with watching TV versus reading. In both cases, the subjects were reclining and completely inactive. It was assumed that the calorie burn for both activities would be the same as resting metabolism.

The readers' metabolisms stayed at the basal level, as expected, but get this: *Television watchers actually had their metabolisms go down by up to 16%!* That's enough to pack on a few pounds per year for the average viewer.

The lower metabolism is thought to be caused by our brains shutting down during TV. Under normal circumstances, a brain burns a lot of calories throughout the day—about 450—but apparently only if you keep it engaged.

The takeaway message: now you really can't justify munching on snacks while watching TV. How about some ab crunches instead?

Another Great Idea that Didn't Work

It's official. Another great weight-loss idea has backfired.

This time it's the 100-calorie-snack-packs of cookies, crackers and other treats. Recent studies show that people tend to eat *more* calories throughout the day when they include these foods in their diet.

How can this be?!

Apparently these single-serving treats feel so harmless that they don't get picked up by our personal "guilt radar." Experts believe that eating treats normally makes you compensate by eating healthier later on. The small-serving snack-packs don't.

I am especially convinced that this is true with children. When I ask kids to name healthy foods, they frequently mention Oreo snack-packs or Goldfish snack-packs right along with the fruits and veggies.

I think these snack packs can still be a good idea—
just make sure to tell your kids or yourself that it's
still junk.

Jill's Favorite Functional Flight Foods

Flying is hard on your body for many reasons—it can leave you dehydrated, constipated, exposed to extra germs and radiation, not to mention stressed. Here are a few tricks for protecting yourself:

1) Carry green, red or white tea bags

The antioxidants help protect you from the extra radiation at high altitudes and, of course, these kinds of tea are hydrating. Get some hot water after you pass through security and enjoy your tea before, during or right after your flight.

2) Garlic

Approximately 20% of travelers catch a cold after flying, so eating this natural germ-killer (ideally raw) is a small price to pay for prevention. Try putting 2 cloves of crushed garlic in some salsa, bruschetta or any other meal right before or after you fly.

3) Walnuts

The omega-3 fatty acids help keep your stress level down, and the usual nut-quantity-problem (so hard to stop at just one serving!) is avoided because you'll only pack 1 ounce to begin with. Eat nuts in place of starches on a flight because you don't need the carbs when you are so sedentary.

4) Bran-a-Crisp Crackers

Eat a couple of these with plenty of water and they will not only fill you up, but also solve any post-flight constipation problems. You can find them at Whole Foods, Gelson's or my office.

5) Cottage Cheese and Frozen Berries

This makes a great travel snack because the protein keeps your metabolism up and the frozen berries keep the whole thing cool for hours.

Happy Travels!

Baker's Demise

At the risk of sounding like the Grinch, I have a cautionary tale for you:

Last year my husband and I made a few teensy-tiny chocolate chip cookies. We only made 8, knowing we'd eat as many as we made. We used a banana instead of sugar and butter, used oats and oat bran instead of flour, used only the whites of the egg, and added only a few chocolate chips. While gobbling them up, we congratulated ourselves on our healthy choices.

Then we decided to calculate the calories.

Our 8 tiny cookies had 1,200 calories! Even though we had removed the most fattening ingredients, we still had some very caloric little treats.

Lesson: *All* baked goods are calorically dense because unlike fruits, veggies, lean meats or unprocessed grains, they contain very little water.

Suggestion: Instead of baking this holiday season, try making wonderful soups and stews. Research shows that people who eat more broth-based soups eat fewer calories without even trying. Or make garlands out of cranberries and popcorn as a tasty, low-cal way to have fun with your kids.

If this sounds like it's going to suck all the fun out of the holidays, just think how rewarding it will feel come January 1st, when you don't have all that cookie-weight to lose!

Gifts of Health

Why not give (and ask for) holiday gifts that will promote health and fitness all year long? Here are some suggestions.

Jill's Healthiest Gift Ideas

Exercise Gear:

- heart rate monitor
- pedometer
- hand weights
- exercise bands
- exerball
- Bosu ball
- exercise videos
- Camelback water pouch
- exercise clothes
- GPS pedometer
- walkman/iPod
- swimming walkman

- reflective clothing
- rollerblades
- treadmill, stair climber, etc.
- Pilates equipment—mats, reformer, etc.

Gift certificates:

- personal training
- massage
- gym membership
- spa treatments
- healthy cooking lessons
- dancing lessons
- a personal chef for a week

Healthy cooking accessories:

- George Foreman Grill
- popcorn air-popper
- vegetable juicer
- yogurt maker
- grain thermos
- veggie steamer
- tea and tea accessories
- milk foamer
- microwave egg poacher
- automatic egg boiler

- salad spinner

Other items:

- health magazine subscription
- health newsletter subscription
- books, cookbooks
- fruit-of-the-month club
- vegetable-of-the-month club
- spa item-of-the-month club
- Tempurpedic mattress
- body pillow
- massage chair
- air purifier
- small bowls and plates (because you eat less on small dinnerware)

Also, remind your family that you **do not want** to receive chocolates, candy or any other unhealthy gifts.

Fall Back into Exercise

Daylight Savings Time ends soon, and that extra hour makes it the perfect time to start a morning exercise habit. Did you know...

1) Morning exercisers are less likely to miss workouts than evening exercisers.

2) Morning exercise gives your metabolism a nice boost for the day.

3) There is less air pollution early in the day.

4) Your body chemistry is best for burning fat and building muscle in the morning (because cortisol levels are highest, which mobilizes fat and sugar into your bloodstream).

With all these incentives *plus* an extra hour, you are out of excuses *not* to exercise. And if you already have this wonderful habit, enjoy your well-deserved extra sleep!

Shoes to Lose

Did you know that the type of shoes you typically wear can affect your weight? In a study of daily physical activity, people were more active when they were wearing more comfortable, less formal shoes. But here's the best part—they weren't *trying* to be more active, and they weren't even *aware* of it! So try putting away the stilettos and see if some pounds come off.

Potatoes Not Prozac

Here's a neat trick for next time you need to feel a bit more happy and relaxed, especially to fall asleep at night. Kathleen DesMaison's book, "Potatoes Not Prozac", shows how the right food combination and timing can act like a dose of Prozac. Here's how:

Eat lean animal protein and let the meal digest for a couple of hours, which will put the amino acid tryphtophan in your blood stream. Then, if you eat half a plain baked potato (or 100 calories of any high-glycemic carbohydrate), the insulin you produce will carry the tryphtophan into the brain, where it gets turned into serotonin, the neurochemical that makes you feel calm, sleepy and content.

For example, try eating chicken plus veggies at dinner and then eat half of a plain potato 2 hours later. See if that helps you feel ready for bedtime.

I was skeptical at first, but I think it worked on me and I've since witnessed hundreds of clients get good results. The trick is to have the self-control to not overeat those carbs. 100 calories is the amount that will give you the effect without going overboard and storing fat.

Food Combining Fads

There are lots of myths about food combining, most of which have never been proven with scientific research. Here are some of the few combinations with evidence to back them up. You'll see there aren't many.

The Good Combinations:

1) Lemon in your green tea boosts the antioxidant effect.

2) Vitamin C-rich foods with iron-rich foods boosts iron absorption.

3) Veggies with a little healthy fat (like olive oil) help you absorb fat-soluble vitamins.

The Bad Combinations:

1) Milk in your tea reduces the heart-healthy benefits.

2) Iron-rich foods with calcium-rich foods blocks absorption of both minerals.

It is also common for people to have their own personal food combination preferences. Listen to your body, but don't listen to the hype that comes from unproven fad diets.

The Mind-Mouth Gap

Here's a funny, depressing, but fixable statistic: According to the September Berkeley Wellness Letter, we Americans are terrible at accurately remembering what we put in our mouths. They report that the average person underestimates their food intake by 800 calories per day.

Whoa! That's enough to pack on the pounds and hamper the best intentions for weight loss. It only takes 3500 excess calories to make a pound of fat.

This helps explain why people who measure and record their food get much better results. If you are struggling to lose weight, get out your measuring cup and recommit to your food journal...at least for a few days to make sure you aren't mis-estimating your way to failure.

Be especially mindful of the calorie-dense foods like oils, butter, nuts, cheese and baked goods. These foods can add loads of calories in just a few easily-forgotten bites.

Salt Solutions

Do you sometimes eat chips, fries, pretzels and the like because you're craving salt? Well, stop it! You don't need to eat fatty, high-carb, processed junk if all you're craving is salt. Here are some quick snacks that give you salt without all that other bad stuff:

- pickles (3 calories each)
- Hearts of Palm (10 calories each)
- canned artichoke hearts (60 calories per 15 oz can)
- Sea's Gift Seaweed snack (20 calories for the smaller package)
- sliced water chestnuts with salt sprinkled on top (100 calories per cup)
- cucumber slices with salt and herbs (negligible calories)
- ...or how about just adding salt or salsa to your salad or steamed veggies?

Don't let a salt craving become a junk food fest when salty *healthy* foods will satisfy.

80 Can Be the New 40

This Wednesday is the 80th birthday of Joyce Ruygrok, the Founder of Diet for Health. If you know Joyce, you know she is physically and mentally more youthful than most of us and still has the knockout figure from when she was a Goldwyn Girl in the 1940's.

True to character, she is spending her birthday week taking care of her daughter (back surgery), throwing an all-night party for her grandson (3am Batman movie with a dozen teenagers) and spending hours playing Nintendo (Wii Fitness, no less!).

How does she do it?!

You can take heart in the fact that it's not just genetic luck. I've seen her mediocre metabolism (about 1200 calories/day) and she has to work at her fitness, just like the rest of us!

Here are some of her secrets:

1) Joyce makes a splurge plan. With her active social life and travel schedule, Joyce always looks ahead to what special treats she wants to save up for. That helps her willpower in the interim.

2) Joyce weighs herself each morning and especially right after she returns from a trip. It might sound obsessive, but research shows this helps people maintain their weight better.

3) Joyce gives tirelessly and finds the good in everything. Joyce spends more hours volunteering than most of us spend working! There is conclusive evidence that volunteerism, optimism and having a life's purpose are great for health and longevity. In addition to making the world a better place, they help keep you from eating out of boredom, stress or loneliness.

4) Joyce follows the Diet for Health menus when she's at home—which isn't very often—and watches her portions otherwise.

Joyce is proof that a little hard work can make 80 the new 40.

Thanks for inspiring us, Joyce!

The Swimming/Fat Burning Mystery

If you like to swim, it's good to be familiar with the Swim/Fat mystery. No, it's not a Nancy Drew novel, but a conundrum about why swimming doesn't seem to help average people lose weight.

I know—it sounds crazy! Swimming uses so many muscles at once, and it sure feels like hard work. Alas, research shows that while swimming is excellent for your heart, muscles and joints, it doesn't take off the pounds as well as other forms of exercise.

Some possible explanations and solutions are:

1) Swimming doesn't get your heart rate high enough, since the smaller muscles of your arms are doing almost all of the work. To fix this, you can buy fins, large or small, that give your legs a killer workout and raise your heart rate.

2) The water and horizontal body position makes it easier for your heart to pump blood than when you

are on land fighting gravity. To remedy this, just swim faster.

3) Most people just get too relaxed in the water and don't push themselves hard enough.

4) Swimming—especially in colder water—increases your appetite. Studies show that people eat about 30% more calories after swimming in a cold pool than in a very warm one.

Whatever the reason, keep swimming! Just try pushing yourself a little harder and make sure you don't overeat afterwards. And don't be surprised if you need to add some other forms of exercise to really see the pounds come off.

Five Pounds of Filling Food

Did you know that most people consume about five pounds of food each day? That's how much food it takes to make the average person feel satisfied. Studies show that the best way to lose weight is to eat bulky, heavy, low-calorie foods so that when you reach your five pounds you haven't eaten too many calories.

What are the heavy, low-calorie foods? You guessed it—they're the ones that are high in (heavy but calorie-free) fiber and water:

- vegetables (about 90% water and fiber)
- fruits (about 80%)
- broth-based soups (95%)

That's why people lose more weight the more they bulk up on these foods and avoid processed foods, where the water and fiber has been removed. It makes sense—you'd have to eat about 10 cups of broccoli to get the calories in one waterless, fiberless ounce of crackers. And a giant salad is just a big pile of water and fiber. Mmm.....is your mouth watering?

Weekend Weakness

The weekend is never far off, and for most people that means fun, relaxation and poor food choices. On average, Americans eat 500-1000 calories more on weekend days than on weekdays **without realizing it**! Those calories add up fast—you'd have to walk about 10-20 extra miles per weekend to work that off—so be mindful about your weekend food choices.

Be especially mindful on long weekends, like the Fourth of July. Make plans now to get active and have healthy options for your holiday festivities. Your weekend does **not** need to revolve around fattening food! How about an Independence Day hike? Or re-enact Paul Revere's famous horseback ride! How about a Boston **green** tea party?

Whatever you do, remember that weekends are the most important time to watch your food intake. Monday morning will feel a whole lot better if you do.

Summer Snacks

Summer is here, so eat these super-foods while they are in season:

- gazpacho soup (keep it handy as an anytime snack)
- mango slices (with cinnamon, perhaps)
- corn on the cob (if you consider it a grain instead of a veggie, it's super nutritious)
- berries and cherries (the fountain of youth and cherries fight pain)
- grape tomatoes
- red peppers (they travel well as snacks; slice them ahead of time, or just bring the entire pepper plus a paring knife)
- papaya with lime
- portabella mushrooms (grill them like hamburgers)
- watermelon (sprinkle cocoa powder and stevia on top and it tastes like fudge cake)
- anything else you find at the farmer's market

...well *almost* anything you find at the farmers market. When it comes to Kettle Korn and candied nuts, enjoy your free sample and don't even *think* of buying any!

A Nutty Solution

If you are trying to lose weight, you are probably struggling with "The Nut Problem": you know that nuts are nutritious, tasty and convenient, but you also know that a quarter cup serving has about 200 calories. Yikes!

Here's one solution: almond milk.

Almond milk tastes great and has only half the calories of nonfat milk. Almond Breeze, the most common brand (at Whole Foods and Trader Joe's) is a fabulous caloric bargain:

- Original unsweetened has 40 calories per cup
- Vanilla unsweetened has 45
- Chocolate unsweetened has 45

All without the hormones that often accompany dairy. The main ingredients are almonds, water and added calcium.

April Foolin'

April Fool's Day is an appropriate time to remind you to *always consider the source* of any nutrition information before you accept it as true. Food and supplement companies have huge financial incentives to exaggerate or even mislead you about their products, and unfortunately the FDA does not have the authority or resources to make sure all claims are true.

Vitamin and herbal supplements are especially known for making dubious claims. Independent testing laboratories have found that many supplements don't contain the amounts of ingredients listed on the label and, even if they do, most are not proven to be safe and effective. Recent tests have also found that herbs and supplements from China sometimes contain scary contaminants, such as heavy metals and even prescription drugs.

You can generally trust nutrition information that comes from respected institutions, such as well-known universities and medical journals. Be especially suspicious of health information that comes from someone who stands to profit from it—like the manufacturer or seller of the item.

Remember that testimonials are often used to sell products that don't pass scientific muster.

When the truly miraculous health and weight loss supplement is discovered, it won't be a secret for long. Our doctors, health insurance companies and political leaders will be quick to get us using any cure that helps us see results. Until then, good old exercise and healthy eating are the only sure bets.

Happy April Fool's Day!

Spend Your Willpower Wisely

As Easter approaches (or *Feaster*, for some) it helps to focus your willpower where it will help most. So remember this: *a single pig-out is not as bad as a bad habit*. Why? It takes 3500 excess calories to gain a pound of fat. Even in your most indulgent feast you probably couldn't eat nearly that much. That's the good news. The bad news is that if you habitually overeat by only 9 calories per day you'll gain a pound of fat by the end of the year. In fact, the average American overeats by 19 calories per day, which is why they gain 20 pounds per decade—yikes!!

Knowing this, put your willpower in the right place. Enjoy a holiday indulgence if you like, but make darn sure that you return to some squeaky clean good habits come Monday morning. The day-in day-out eating practices are what make or break you, not the occasional treat. Happy Easter!

Spring Forward

Daylight Savings Time is finally here, and it's the perfect time to start a wonderful habit:

Get active after dinner!

This will make a big difference to your health and weight loss because:

1) Physical activity helps reduce post-meal blood sugar spikes, which contribute to fat storage,

2) After dinner is the most sedentary time of day for most people, and

3) After dinner is when the most junk food gets eaten (and you can't eat junk if you're outside having fun, right?).

So get out there and walk around the neighborhood, play with your dog, throw a Frisbee or just get out and enjoy summer. You'll be amazed what a difference it makes!

Protein Problems

Uh oh! America is doing it again. We're thinking that portions don't matter so long as we eat the right type of food—in this case protein. In the 1980's we made the same mistake with carbs—remember when we thought we could eat unlimited bagels and SnackWell Cookies because they had no fat? Those were the days...until we gained weight and type 2 diabetes, anyway.

Here's why gorging on protein is not OK:

1) Protein has 4.5 calories per gram, the same as carbohydrate, and excess calories from any source will be stored as fat.

2) When you metabolize protein for fuel, it creates waste products that your kidneys must excrete. Too much protein can lead to kidney strain or damage. New findings from China show that people eating less animal protein tend to have better health and live longer.

The conflict is that animal protein aids weight loss because it is more satisfying and filling than carbs or fat and it also boosts your metabolism. What is a person to do?

Eat moderate amounts of protein and then load up on veggies!

Overeating of VEGETABLES is so far undocumented, and research suggests that your health and weight **improve** the more you eat.

Soy Story

If you don't want a double chin with that soymilk mustache, make sure to check the nutrition label.

Not all soymilks are created equal. They range from 60 to 210 calories per cup! Some have loads of added sugar, but even very natural ones (just soy and water) can be high in fat because of the natural fat in the soybean. The best for weight loss is Vitasoy Light Original. It has the fewest calories (60), fat (2g) and sugar (4g) of any I've seen. The most nutritious are the ones with the fewest ingredients—just soybeans and water. The same goes for rice milk and almond milk.

Also, remember that the soymilks used at Starbucks and other cafes are usually the tastiest ones, which are high in sugar. Nonfat milk is a better choice at Starbucks if you are watching calories and sugar.

Better than Water

I, your trusty nutritionist, don't drink much water. That's because I believe there are lots of things that hydrate you as well (or better) and which also come packed with lots of natural nutrients. New research is showing that getting nutrients in their natural form (as opposed to in man-made supplements) is very important, so here are my favorite ways to hydrate without water:

- green tea
- white tea
- red tea
- the water left over when you steam veggies
- low-sodium veggie soup
- fresh vegetables

Vegetables?! Yes! It turns out that these foods are mostly water with lots of vitamins and minerals attached. That means your big salad is practically a big plate of electrolyte-enhanced water...with a whole bunch of healthy fiber added!

Fat-Burning Date Nights

Here are some ideas for non-fattening ways to enjoy an evening out because the customary "stuff and sit" outings—where you overeat and then let it all turn to fat as you watch a show—lead to regret on Monday morning!

1) Go dancing or take dance lessons.

2) Go for a hike.

3) Have a healthy picnic and play Frisbee.

4) Get spa treatments together.

5) Have a Shabu Shabu or broth fondue dinner at home or at your favorite Shabu restaurant.

6) Go ice skating or rollerskating (Moonlight Roller Rink in Burbank has themed music nights and evenings reserved for skaters over 30).

7) Play mini-golf.

8) Take a yoga or Pilates class.

9) Enjoy a messy meal pulling fresh crab or lobster out of its shell (no butter sauce!).

10) For the truly adventurous...take trapeze lessons! There is a circus school in Hollywood where anybody can learn.

Consider making these part of your weekend routine and please share your favorite healthy activities that I failed to mention!

Good Willpower Hunting

We could all use a little extra willpower this time of year, so it's a good time to review the things you can do to help strengthen it:

1) Get enough sleep (7+ hours for most people).

2) Minimize stress.

3) Prevent low blood sugar by eating small snacks every few hours.

4) Pamper yourself with non-edible treats, like bubble baths, massage, etc.

Research shows that these things make a big difference! Give it a try and remember that the best strategy is to minimize your dependence on willpower by getting all tempting treats out of your home ASAP!

Thanksgiving Tips

Here are 10 ways to make your Thanksgiving Day a little healthier. Do at least 3 of these and I'll be very thankful!

1) Eat a healthy breakfast on Thanksgiving morning (it prevents overeating later).

2) Get some exercise.

3) Be the slowest eater at the table. Set your fork down between every bite of food.

4) Drink lots of water the whole day through and have small snacks when you get hungry.

5) Eat your turkey and healthiest veggies first, before you eat the stuffing, potatoes, etc.

6) Go for a walk after dinner (it helps prevent your blood sugar from rising too high too fast).

7) Remember the 3-bite rule: 90% of the flavor is in the first 3 bites. That means you don't need a huge slice of pie!

8) Give away the most unhealthy leftovers.

9) Have healthy meals and a good workout planned for the day after Thanksgiving, to get right back on track.

10) Take a moment to be thankful and to enjoy your family and friends. I'm not being sentimental— research shows that this can improve your health!

Have a very happy Thanksgiving!

Fat-Burning Factoids

Now we're starting Holiday Weight-Gain Season, so here are a few of the latest research findings on how to prevent holiday heft:

1) People who eat breakfast consume about 5% fewer calories over the course of the day. That's about 100 calories, which adds up to losing over 10 pounds per year!

2) New studies are finding that cortisol—the stress hormone—interferes with the transmission of leptin, the "satisfaction" hormone that tells you to stop eating. This explains why you are hungrier when you're stressed. Try to manage stress and be extra conscientious about watching your portion sizes when things get hectic.

3) Saturated fat—the kind in cheese, cream, butter, beef (i.e. fat from any animal except fish)—does not trigger the release of leptin as much as healthy fats like nuts or olive oil. That means you get less satisfaction and "fullness" from these unhealthy fats.

The Great Pumpkin

With Halloween coming soon, it's time to spread the word to all parents about **The Great Pumpkin.**

Monica DeMoulin, a health-conscious mother of two, came up with this fabulous idea. Here's how it works: The day after Halloween, kids choose their very favorite 10-20 pieces of candy that they have collected. They leave the rest for The Great Pumpkin, who will come during the night and take the candy for children who don't have any. In return, The Great Pumpkin (i.e. mom or dad) leaves a toy or gift for the child. The more candy the child leaves, the nicer the gift that The Great Pumpkin leaves behind!

This works really well—kids love it!—so give it a try and spread the word. All kids (even the skinniest ones) are better off not eating all that sugar.

p.s. If you are an adult with a sweet tooth, feel free to be your own Great Pumpkin. Bribery is better than a sugar binge any day.

Halloween Haunts 'til New Year

Here's a haunting statistic: The average American gains 4-8 pounds between Halloween and New Year's Day. Yikes!

The first step toward prevention is ***don't spike your blood sugar on Halloween***!

Many people find that a single sugar binge can throw off your body chemistry and cause:

1) greater sugar cravings

2) increased appetite

3) weaker willpower

You can't afford to have that happen just as the holiday season starts...you're going to need to be at your best to weather all the holiday parties and treats coming your way until January!

So spend this Halloween bobbing for apples, toasting pumpkin seeds or spooking your friends, but don't go crazy on candy! If you ***do*** go crazy on candy, make sure to throw away your leftovers so that it can't become a habit.

p.s. Sugar-free candy won't spike your blood sugar, but remember that it's often not as low-calorie as you might think. Read the label.

Chilling and Cheating

Happy Autumn!

It's a good time to know that recent studies confirm what we Northerners have long suspected: Being cold makes you hungry.

In one study, people consumed 30% more calories at a meal when they had recently been subjected to cold. That's a lot of extra calories! So bundle up this winter, and if you do happen to get cold, be extra mindful of what you eat afterwards. Keep hot tea and hot brothy soups on hand, and feel free to use this as justification for a few more long, hot bubble baths!

Food and Acne

While research has never supported the old wive's tale that grease or chocolate causes acne, it has recently found a diet-complexion connection. While some acne is caused purely by bacteria or hormones, there is also a dietary culprit. It is...drum roll please...

High-glycemic foods!

These are the processed foods that raise your blood sugar quickly, often causing an insulin surge. High-glycemic foods include:

- almost everything made from white flour: bread, pastries, pretzels, muffins, cereal
- almost everything high in sugar: soda, candy, cookies, cake
- most processed foods

You should already be avoiding high-glycemic foods because they contribute to weight gain, diabetes, mood swings, high triglycerides and have poor nutritional value. But now, as if that weren't enough, they've also been shown to promote acne.

Losing Over Labor Day

Researchers have estimated that the average person eats 500-1000 extra calories on weekend days...without even realizing it. Yikes!

Given that we have a *long* holiday weekend coming, it pays to make a plan for getting through it without gaining weight:

1) Figure out what super-healthy breakfast you can eat (egg white omelet with veggies and salsa?) in anticipation of extra treats tempting you later in the day.

2) What healthy snacks can you bring with you to parties? Crudite and shrimp cocktail are perfect, easy options.

3) Should you eat a salad or an apple before going out?

4) Can you fit in an extra workout over the weekend? How about a few extra hours of sleep?

5) Remember the 3 Bite Rule: 90% of the pleasure of any food comes in the first 3 bites.

Make your plan *right now* so you'll have time to prepare. You'll be glad you did!

Intensity is IN!

If you don't have much time for exercise, there's good news. Lots of new research is finding that intensity—even more than duration—is important for most benefits to health and fitness. For example, intensity is more valuable than time spent exercising when it comes to:

1) longevity—intense exercise makes your cells act younger

2) metabolism—you get a longer "afterburn"

3) speed and performance

4) heart health

Try interval training for shorter and more effective workouts. Just make sure to get your doctor's OK and warm up first. The intense intervals can be as short as 8 seconds or as long as 2 minutes, with a slower pace afterwards until your heart rate recovers, usually 1-5 minutes.

Try it twice per week and see how fast your fitness improves! If you are a bootcamper or take my cardio-sculpt class at Caltech, congrats! You are already interval training.

Food Fabrication

You may have never asked the question "What is food made of?", but the answer will change the way you think about and choose foods.

All foods have varying amounts of:

1) Fat

2) Protein

3) Carbohydrates

4) Fiber

5) Water

6) Vitamins and minerals

7) Additives (if the food has been processed with them)

Americans these days are eating too much of ingredients 1-3 (where all the calories are) and not enough of 4-6, which is why Americans are called "overfed but undernourished." How do you get more of the good stuff while cutting down on the other? It's easy and not surprising: eat more fruits, veggies, whole grains and lean meats. These foods are naturally high in water, fiber, vitamins and minerals, which is why they are more filling per calorie than other foods.

Processed foods generally have the least water, fiber, vitamins and minerals because these things are removed or destroyed during processing. For the next few days try thinking of your food as the components that make it and see how it affects your choices. For example, a salad is just a big pile of water, fiber and nutrients!

Is your mouth watering?

Outing Inflammation

Diet-related inflammation is a hot topic these days because it affects both health and beauty—it causes tissue to become red and puffy, which isn't healthy *or* attractive!

Inflammation most commonly contributes to joint pain, cardiovascular damage and a ruddy complexion. Here's how food works in:

Inflammatory Foods:

- white flour
- sugar
- salt
- high-fat beef
- high-fat dairy
- anything highly processed (even bread and breakfast cereal)

Anti-Inflammatory Foods:

- nuts (especially walnuts)
- seeds (especially flax)

- green, white or red tea
- berries (any kind)
- olive oil
- salmon, tuna, other fatty fish
- all colorful vegetables

This is a great way to eat for health *and* weight loss, so long as you don't overdo the healthy fats (remember, a serving of nuts or seeds is only 1/4 cup and a serving of oil is only 1 Tbsp.). If you have arthritis, Rosacea, heart disease or just want radiant skin, give this a try and see if you look and feel better.

Vacation Vexation

In my experience, people don't blow their diet **on** vacation as much as they do upon **returning from** vacation!

When you get back from vacation, you are swamped with mail, phone messages, etc. and there is nothing to eat in the house, right? Here's an easy solution: Plan your menu for your first day back before you even leave. For example, stock the kitchen with:

- frozen veggies and protein for making a quick stir-fry dinner

- oats and frozen berries for breakfast

- egg beaters and frozen veggies for a quick omelet

- cans of tuna, healthy soups, wasa crackers or other convenience foods from our "favorite foods shelf"

- a grocery list of everything (especially fresh fruits and veggies) that you should buy ASAP

It pays to get right back to your good habits the **minute** you return because then you don't give any bad habits a chance to take hold. Think of it as throwing yourself a healthy "welcome home" party!

Sleep Matters

We all know that sleep makes us feel great, but new research shows that only 2 nights of sleep deprivation (defined as 4 hours of sleep) changes your body's hormonal chemistry to:

1) increase your appetite

2) impede your satiety signals (that means it takes more food to make you feel full)

3) cause carbohydrate cravings

Even if you get more than 4 hours of sleep regularly, a small sleep deficit may add up over time, so *make sleep a priority* if you are trying to lose weight!

Now isn't that better than having to exercise more?

Sweet (and Juicy) Success

Ever since the low-carb fad came along, many folks have avoided fruit because it contains sugar. Well, new research proves that fruit is a sweet and juicy way to stay slim! A new study has concluded that frequent fruit eaters experience less weight gain over time compared to people who report low fruit consumption. Fresh fruit is high in fiber and low in calories, especially for how filling it is.

So stop feeling guilty about fruit and ENJOY!

Junk Food Justified

I'm just back from running the Inca Trail to Machu Picchu and boy, what an experience! Exercising all day at high altitude requires the 4 big sports performance enhancers:

1) salt

2) water

3) high-glycemic carbs

4) caffeine

...in other words, lots of the tasty processed foods you can't normally justify!

Crackers, energy bars, granola bars, pretzels, energy drinks, candy, bread, and chocolate-covered espresso beans are all good ways to get quick energy when you're in the middle of serious endurance exercise. You actually need low-fiber, high-calorie foods at this time because they are fast and easy to digest. Your stomach isn't too good at digesting high-fiber foods when your muscles are using up most of your blood and oxygen.

Enjoy these junky foods during long bouts of exercise because after you recover, it's time to get back to the fresh fruits, veggies, whole grains, lean proteins and unprocessed foods that are full of nutrients and fiber.

Texture Tips

Often when we enjoy a food, it isn't the taste we like so much as the texture. For example, potato chips and pretzels are little more than salt flavor made crunchy. Why eat extra fat, sugar and unwanted calories if it's just the texture you want?! Think about the textures you enjoy in your foods and come up with some *healthy* ways to get them.

For example...

For crunchy snacks try:

- cucumber slices
- jicama
- water chestnut slices
- dill pickles
- hearts of palm
- baby carrots
- baby snap peas
- kale chips (bake de-veined kale leaves at 350 for 10 min and add seasoning if you want them to be salty or spicey)

For smooth, creamy snacks try:

- nonfat yogurt
- nonfat pudding (sugar free is also available)
- pureed fruit (like applesauce)

For frozen treats try:

- a healthy home-made smoothie
- popsicles
- fudgesicles
- carbo-lite frozen yogurt
- no-sugar-added, fat-free blended coffee drinks (Coffee Bean makes the only ones I know of)

Please let me know if you have other ideas for good texture substitutes.

Splurge Scourge

Everybody knows it's healthier to spread out your caloric intake over the entire day with frequent small meals, but many people still prefer to save up most of their calories for a big indulgence once a day or week.

Here's why that makes you gain weight:

An average body can handle at the very most 800 calories at once, and every calorie above that gets turned to fat (it's less if you are small and inactive). So no matter how much you starve yourself before that big dinner, you'll still store fat if you eat (or drink!) more than 800 calories.

Unfortunately it's **extremely** easy to reach 800 calories at a restaurant or any time you consume alcohol or dessert with a meal. The good news is that if you are eating frequent, small meals throughout the day you won't want to overindulge so much at dinner.

Salsa Solution

Are you feeling like your salads, fish, poultry, veggies and whole grains have become more boring than the last hour of traffic school? (Yes, I did traffic school this weekend, so it's salient!) Well then it's time to rediscover salsa!

Salsa has tons of flavor for only about 5 calories per tablespoon because of the zesty (and nutritious) spices. In addition to mild or spicy, there are exotic salsas like mango, ginger or grapefruit. Find a few you like and use them to flavor just about everything. We have recipes at the office, or just use Google. And please share your favorite recipes with us!

When in Rome

Ever wonder how Italians remain slim? Well I don't know how they do it, but they must not be eating in *our* Italian restaurants!

The average plate of pasta in an American Italian restaurant is up to 3.5 cups—that's 7 servings and 700 calories *before* they even add any sauce—yikes! Here are some tips for eating out Italian:

1) Don't let the bread basket sit near you (don't even let it on the table if your tablemates are willing).

2) Get salad or minestrone soup for an appetizer.

3) Look for seafood, chicken or salad dishes on the menu. Ask for dressings and sauces on the side.

4) Avoid cheese and Alfredo sauce (the original "heart attack on a plate").

5) Ask for the "to go" box right away and put half of your meal in there before you even start eating.

6) *Need* pasta? Ask for a child-size portion in addition to your soup or salad.

7) *Need* pizza or calzone? Ask for a cheeseless version with lots of veggies and chicken. Restaurants will always be able to accommodate you (they get

plenty of demands for cheeseless pizza from people who are lactose intolerant).

8) Instead of wine, how about that fancy Italian bottled water?

Making Mexican

Now for tips on another most fattening ethnic meal out: Mexican.

Tip 1: Order your meal without the cheese! When you eat full-fat cheese, you might as well just paste it to your rear and block off some arteries.

Tip 2: Lose the sour cream, guacamole and chips.

Tip 3: If you must eat tortilla chips, slow yourself down by breaking each one into a dozen or so mini-pieces. Make yourself eat one mini-piece at a time.

Very Best Choices:

- tostada salad with chicken (but skip the 800-calorie fried tortilla shell)
- chicken fajitas
- any taco or burrito that has mostly lean meat, veggies, lettuce, tomato and salsa (but keep in mind that a single burrito-size tortilla has about 450 calories, so try not to eat the whole thing!)

Good luck, and remember the two most important words in the Mexican restaurant language: "sin quesa."

Rack the Thai

Thai food is so delicious...but my clients almost always gain weight after eating at a Thai restaurant. Here are some ways to enjoy it without the damage:

Tip 1: Try to go to a more upscale Thai restaurant, where healthier dishes are easier to come by.

Tip 2: Order the simpler meals on the menu so that you know exactly what ingredients are in your food. Avoid anything fried or swimming in coconut milk, peanut sauce or curry.

Tip 3: Get an order of steamed veggies on the side.

Tip 4: The healthiest Thai food I know of in our area is at Saladang Song in Pasadena.

Best choices:

- broth-based soups containing veggies, chicken or seafood
- stir-fries containing lots of veggies, chicken or shrimp
- salads with the dressing on the side
- simpler fish, chicken or seafood dishes

Stress Busting

I hope this finds you without too much stress in your life, but if it does, here are some things you can do:

1) Eat fish, nuts and seeds daily. Salmon, tuna, walnuts and flax seeds are especially good. The healthy fats in these foods help boost mood and prevent anxiety.

2) Don't skip meals or snacks. When things get stressful you mustn't forget to eat. Low blood sugar will worsen your mood and your ability to cope.

3) Exercise the stress hormones away. If you let adrenaline and cortisol build up in your body, they age you and damage your health. When you exercise, you use them up and they actually *help* you burn fat!

4) Don't turn to comfort food for relief. Yes, it calms you, but you'll be sorry later! Be strong and try relaxing with laughter, massage or a bubble bath instead.

Timing is Everything

Did you know that timing is everything when it comes to eating for best energy, metabolism, muscle-building and fat burning?

It is best to eat proportionally to how much energy you are burning at the time. That means if you are burning the most energy in the morning and being sedentary all evening, you should eat the most calories in the morning and eat light in the evening. *This is the biggest mistake I see people make*—they don't eat too much, they just time it wrong and consume all their calories at night when they burn most of their calories earlier in the day.

You may need to wake up earlier to make time for a bigger breakfast and to pack some snacks for the day. You'll also need to resist the urge to reward yourself at the end of the day with a big meal (unless you plan to be very active in the evening.) These changes are tough at first, but will make all the difference in the end.

Sleep and Eating: Mystery Solved!

You already know that sleep deprivation contributes to hunger, cravings and weight gain, but new research shows why. It has to do with 2 hormones that regulate appetite: grehlin, which stimulates hunger and leptin, which suppresses appetite. I bet you can guess what researchers found. People who slept fewer than 5 hours per night had more ghrelin and less leptin than people who had 8 hours sleep or more.

This makes sleep one of the most important (and painless!) parts of your weight loss efforts.

Salad Savvy

Here's a research tidbit you can use: researchers had 42 women eat as much pasta as they wanted for lunch, with or without a salad first. If the women ate a salad with only veggies and low-cal dressing, they ate 12% fewer calories overall than eating the pasta alone. No big surprise.

Here's the surprise: if they first ate a calorie-dense salad (with regular dressing and cheese), then they ended up eating many *more calories than if they ate only pasta!*

Moral of the story: either stick with low-cal salad ingredients or don't bother eating salads at all!

Try flavoring your salads with salsa, fresh fruit, a variety of veggies and vinegars and you'll have plenty of flavor.

Biology of Bingeing, Part I

If you have seen the documentary "March of the Penguins", then you have seen why gorging on huge quantities of food has historically been a valuable habit for survival.

In the movie we see that each year the Emperor Penguins walk (with very small, clumsy steps!) over 70 miles to their breeding ground, where they will court and mate. After laying an egg, the female will walk back 70 miles to the ocean to feed while the male stays behind to incubate the egg, trying to keep himself and the egg warm for 4 months of frigid cold and Antarctic storms. He can't eat during that time and is near starvation by the time the baby penguin hatches. If all goes well, the mother returns with a belly full of food to share with the chick, and the male walks back 70 miles (nearly starved) to the ocean to refill his belly. If the mother shows up too late, the chick will starve or the father will be forced to return to the ocean (leaving the chick to die) because he needs to eat or he will die.

Starvation is constantly a threat.

Now try to imagine a penguin who, during her brief feeding opportunity says "Goodness, I think I'm satisfied on a small quantity and I don't want to stuff myself." There probably have been such penguins. And they get weeded out of the gene pool very quickly! Only the ones that stuff themselves silly have enough food to survive the long walks and hard living until they will have their next feeding opportunity.

This is one example of why animals are programmed to overeat. Our ancient biology doesn't know that food is plentiful and life is easy. I like to remind myself that rather than feeling guilty about wanting to overeat, I should feel lucky that my ancestors did so, because that's likely the reason my genes survived this long.

Overeating is natural, so we shouldn't feel guilty—but that doesn't mean we shouldn't use smart strategies for avoiding it. I'll write more about that tomorrow. In the meantime, let your conscience be clear about overeating and blame your biology.

Beating Overeating (Part 2)

If you love to eat and sometimes struggle with stopping, here are some interesting research tidbits that help.

Strategies to help prevent overeating:

1) Minimize side dishes.

The more food choices you have, the more you eat. Studies show that when you have only 1 or 2 dishes in front of you, you eat less food overall than if you have 3 or 4 choices. This means you need to be extra careful at buffets and potlucks.

2) Use music to your advantage.

Listen to mellow music at mealtime. A study at Johns Hopkins University found that diners chew faster and eat more when listening to lively music and eat less with relaxing music.

3) Dim the lights.

Another study at Johns Hopkins found that diners ate less food under low lighting.

4) Use smaller utensils.

This forces you to take smaller bites and eat more slowly.

5) Get enough sleep.

Well-rested people overeat less, probably because they have fewer cravings and don't need to rely so much on food to keep up their energy level.

6) Be the slowest eater in a group.

The larger the group, the more each person tends to eat—without realizing it. Be aware that group meals lead to overeating and try to be the slowest eater at the table.

Eating is one of life's great pleasures, but overeating ruins the experience by making you feel regret, guilt and physical discomfort. Use a few of these strategies for a week and see if you can get in the habit of eating only until you are satisfied.

I'm sure you can find *new* things to feel guilty about!

Don't Trust the Chef

Ever wonder why the food you make at home doesn't taste as good as the same thing at a restaurant? Even just rice. Or oatmeal. Or a turkey sandwich? How is that possible?

Well, there are two potential answers:

1) The restaurant chef has skills or ingredients you don't. This is often true.

or...

2) The restaurant chef uses more salt, sugar, oil, butter, lard, cream, etc. than you would ever consider proper. This is *more* often true.

I have been astounded by how many professional chefs will not hesitate to use 10+ servings of oil, butter, salt, etc. to make a single serving of food. When "Take Home Chef" (a television show where a 3-star chef comes to your home and helps you prepare dinner) came to my house, the chef used...

2.5 sticks of butter

.5 liter olive oil

1.5 pints of cream

That is thousands of calories of added fat for only 2 dinners!

This explains why diners usually underestimate the calories in their restaurant meals by 50%. It also explains why it's usually easier to lose weight dining in.

Bowled Over

There is some fascinating research on eating habits and containers! Get this:

- People automatically eat and drink less when they use taller, thinner bowls and glasses. Shorter, wider containers give the illusion of less volume, so people eat more from them.

- People eat less candy or chips out of an opaque bowl than out of one that is transparent. Apparently you are more tempted when you have a better view of the contents.

- People eat less candy or snacks out of a bowl when it is less full. The more snacks in the bowl, the more people eat.

- People eat less food off of dark-colored plates than off of white plates. Without realizing it!

So if you tend to overeat, get yourself to Pottery Barn and get the darkest, tallest, skinniest, most opaque bowls, cups and plates you can find!

Power of Prevention

As I sit here with a raging case of Poison Oak, I'm reminded of how some problems are much easier to *prevent* (scratch, scratch) than to *cure!*

This is surprisingly true in the case of weight gain. You might think that losing a pound of fat involves simply burning off the excess calories that you overate in the first place. Not so, unfortunately. *Burning off a pound of fat is much more work than preventing it.*

Recent research is showing that once new fat is stored on your body, it can be reluctant to leave. It may release hormones that increase your appetite and destabilize blood sugar, making it tougher to eat right. In addition, when you burn off the extra fat you are likely to lose some lean tissue along with it, which lowers your metabolism.

This is *not* to say that weight loss is futile! Everybody backslides sometimes, but you'll save yourself some work if you minimize the number of times you let yourself pig out today with plans to burn it off tomorrow.

Leapin' Leptin

Here's a useful new research finding: calories from saturated fats don't raise leptin levels as much as calories from other foods. Leptin is the hormone that makes you feel full and satisfied, so you want the foods you eat to release more, not less.

Alcohol also tends not to release it.

Interesting! This is one more reason to lay off the cheeseburgers and fries.

...like we needed another reason.

Afternoon Energy Boosters

If you are like most people, you sometimes suffer from an afternoon energy slump that leaves you wishing for a siesta. Many people turn to foods full of sugar or caffeine for a quick energy boost, but those are short-term fixes that leave you worse off in the long run. Luckily there are some healthy alternatives.

Spices like ginger, red cayenne pepper and peppermint can raise your metabolism and give you a natural, healthy lift. You can find ginger and peppermint in herbal teas, chewing gums or hard candies. You can also add these spices to your afternoon snack—try adding red pepper to your cottage cheese or hummus (to eat with veggies) and sprinkle ginger on your apple slices.

It works!

Ideal After-Dinner Drink

Here's a simple way to burn a few more calories, according to a recent study: follow your meals with a tall glass of ice water.

In a small study, men and women who drank 2 cups of cold water after a meal temporarily experienced a 30% increase in the rate at which their bodies burned calories. The increased calorie burning was attributed to thermogenesis, a process by which the body burns calories for digestion purposes. It has been estimated that you can burn about 60 extra calories per day this way. That doesn't sound like much, but as a daily habit that adds up to 21,900 calories (or 6 pounds of fat lost) per year!

Cool, eh?

Buffet Brunch Beware

With Easter and Mother's Day coming, it's time to discuss strategies for surviving buffet brunches. They tend to embody everything you don't want to do if you are watching your weight, so the #1 strategy is to avoid them when possible! If that's not an option:

- Don't starve yourself beforehand. Low blood sugar leads to overeating and bad willpower.

- Be the slowest eater there. Chew thoroughly and set down your fork between bites.

- Fill your first plate with veggies, fruits, lean proteins and salad. Fill up on those things.

- Let your second plate be small servings of the less healthy foods that really appeal to you.

- Plan a good walk or exercise session for later in the day.

Finally, in case you were wondering, you **won't** do well by stuffing yourself at brunch and then not eating the rest of the day. Your metabolism, blood sugar, cholesterol and intestines much prefer a few smaller meals.

If you have an Easter egg hunt, don't forget that toys and coins are better egg stuffers than candy!

For Chocoholics

If I had 3 wishes from a magic genie, I'd probably use 1 of them to invent guilt-free chocolate that we could eat all day long! Until that happens, here are some of our clients' favorite alternatives:

1) Canfield's Diet Chocolate Fudge Soda

2) No Sugar Added Fudgesicles

3) Powdered cocoa (no sugar) + Stevia sprinkled on everything from sliced fruit to oatmeal to cottage cheese

4) Small quantities of dark chocolate

5) Fresh fruit dipped in small quantities of melted chocolate

6) Diet hot cocoa

7) Carbo-Lite Frozen Yogurt

8) Cocoa Spice Tea (by Yogi Teas)

9) 3 savored bites of anything you want...after you have thrown away the rest of it!

Please let me know if you have other chocolatey ideas or if you know where I can find that magic genie!

Tune In or Tone Up

A recent Harvard study found that the risk of becoming obese rises by 23% for every 2 hours of daily television viewing...and the average American watches 5 hours! Yikes!

Why not make a deal with yourself? If you **must** watch TV, don't just sit there. Do sit-ups, leg lifts, and other exercises while you watch. Or chop veggies to have on hand as a healthy snack. Incidentally, TV watching is also correlated with dissatisfaction with one's own appearance, even **before** you've gained any weight! Apparently watching those starlets makes us want to be unrealistically thin, even as it makes us fat! How about a good book instead?

How to Gain Fat on 1000 Calories Per Day

Everybody knows it's healthier to spread out your caloric intake over the entire day with frequent small meals, but many people still prefer to save up most of their calories for a big indulgence once a day. Here's why that makes you gain weight:

An average body can handle *at the very most* 800 calories at once and every calorie above that gets turned to fat (it varies by body size, exercise, etc.) So no matter how much you starve yourself before that big dinner, you'll still store fat if you eat (and/or drink!) more than 800 calories. Unfortunately it's *extremely* easy to reach 800 calories at a restaurant or any time you consume alcohol or dessert with a meal. The good news is that if you are eating frequent, small meals throughout the day you won't want to overindulge so much at dinner. Happy light eating!

Strategic Snacking

There's a dangerous threat to your healthy diet lurking out there and you may not even realize it: *Arriving home at the end of a tiring day with an empty stomach and low blood sugar*. It sounds so harmless, but it's not!

This is the evil monster that leads people to overeat at night. It happens for a simple physiological reason—low blood sugar and a tiring day make your willpower weak, so you give in to the powerful pleas of your empty stomach.

Here's a solution: Have a snack 20-30 minutes before you arrive home. It should be a fruit, yogurt, healthy crackers, or something with some complex carbohydrate to get your blood sugar up. Now when you arrive home, your brain *and* your stomach are in a better position to help you eat right.

Training Prevents Complaining

This week I want to remind you that your time is precious, so don't be one of the many poor souls who wastes their time exercising ineffectively! For cardiovascular exercise, effective training means getting in your proper heart rate zone. For weight training, it gets a little more complicated and this is where lots of exercisers waste their time with improper methods. I recommend having at least a few sessions with a Certified Personal Fitness Trainer. It's a bit expensive, but well worth it, since you'll forevermore get better results for every minute of your workout.

Healthy Mother's Day Ideas

Your mom, wife (or YOU, if you are a mother) deserves the gift of great health this Mother's Day, so instead of a big old brunch, where the whole family stuffs themselves and then feels guilty, how about one of these healthy ideas:

1) Have a Mother's Day picnic with mom's favorite healthy foods and a Frisbee to get everyone active.

2) Go for a Mother's Day fat-burning activity like hiking, bowling or mini-golf.

3) Give (or ask for) healthy Mother's Day gifts, like exercise gadgets or gift certificates for a personal training session or massage. And don't forget that some of the best healthy gifts are free—foot massages, back massages or just the promise of some time alone without any parental duties.

Remember—*holidays don't have to be about food!* Finding other forms of celebration—games, activities, outings, etc.—will be fun *and* healthy.

Just Say No

Happy Holidays! If you are getting more holiday stress than holiday cheer this year (and I know many of you are!) try *just saying no* to non-essential holiday obligations. By reducing stress you will also have a much easier time watching your weight over the holidays because stress tends to:

1) increase your appetite

2) exaggerate cravings for sweets and starches

3) interfere with sleep (better sleep means easier weight loss)

4) make your blood sugar levels less stable (making it harder to lose weight)

So *take time* for yourself this season, even if you have to let a few things slide. *Just say no* to holiday obligations that will be more trouble than they are worth. One of the best gifts you can give your friends and family is a happier, healthier, more relaxed *you*!

Too Much of a Good Thing

With all the recent news about how green tea aids weight loss, prevents cancer and protects health, some of us are bound to overdo it sometimes. If you get nauseous or dizzy from your green tea, you may be drinking too much too fast. Try less gulping and more sipping and see if that helps.

Nutrition Bar Blues

I know you don't want to hear this because they are so convenient, but nutrition bars get a big thumbs-down.

Here's why:

1). According to an independent testing laboratory, over half of the 46 bars tested were lying about their nutrition information. They tended to have more sugar, carbs and calories than listed on the nutrition label.

2) Nutrition bars are not filling enough for the calories they provide. For example, you could eat a large salad or a few cups of fruit for the calories in an average bar. This makes many people eat more at their next meal.

If you regularly eat nutrition bars and aren't getting the results you think you deserve, try replacing them with real food snacks like fruit, veggies, cottage cheese, etc. That usually makes a big difference!

Going Anti-Antioxidant

Throw out your mega-dose antioxidant supplements of beta-carotene and vitamins A and E. A very large examination of 86 studies recently found—to the surprise of many—that folks taking large doses of these antioxidants had shortened lifespans. This is counter-intuitive because antioxidants are thought to protect cells from free radicals (a normal by-product of metabolism). Antioxidants in fruits and veggies are known to help prevent cancer and premature aging.

What happened?

This is one more demonstration of man-made nutrition supplements gone wrong. Whereas naturally-occurring antioxidants in fruits and veggies are known to protect cells, the man-made versions in high doses don't have the same effect. It isn't yet known why or how man-made antioxidants affect the body, but for now you are better off without them.

Eating and Depression

I've always wondered how people could enjoy fishing so much and this might explain it. Get this:

The higher the ratio of omega-6 fatty acids compared to omega-3s in your blood, the more likely you are to suffer from depression.

Omega-6 fatty acids are found in vegetable oils used in margarine, baked goods and snack foods. In the western world, consumption of omega-6 oils is 15 to 17 times that of omega-3s, which are found in fish, flaxseed and walnuts.

Ohio State University College of Medicine researchers found that participants suffering from major depression had blood levels of omega-6 that were nearly 18 times as high as their levels of omega-3. Those who didn't have major depression had blood levels of omega-6 that were about 13 times their levels of omega-3s. The study was published online in Psychosomatic Medicine last month.

For a healthier omega-6/omega-3 balance, eat more flax, walnuts and fatty fish including salmon, mackerel or sardines and eat fewer processed foods made with vegetable oil. Fish oil supplements are also thought to help correct an imbalance.

I feel cheerier already!

Earth Day Diet Tip

"Do you want global warming with that?"

Imagine the voice at the drive-thru asking you this question when you order your cheeseburger. Sounds crazy, right? Not according to the United Nations Food and Agriculture Organization. Their 2006 report warns us that our increasing consumption of animal foods (meat and dairy) is taking a heavy toll on the planet.

The problem is that livestock—while delicious—is tough on the environment in at least three different ways. First, they pollute our water, air and soil with manure and methane (a greenhouse gas that is 23 times more potent at trapping heat than carbon dioxide). Second, the corn, soybeans and hay grown for livestock feed requires huge amounts of fertilizer, which generates large amounts of nitrous oxide. Finally, trees and rainforest lands are being sacrificed to create more land for livestock pasture. One extreme example is Brazil, where about 70 percent of onetime forest land is being used as pasture and to grow animal feed.

The UN report concludes that eating less meat and dairy foods is one step we could all take to help reduce global warming and other environmental damage.

Here's the great news: what's good for the planet is also great for your health. Replacing animal foods with plant foods—like fruits, veggies, grains, beans, nuts, seeds, legumes—prevents obesity, heart disease, diabetes, stroke and cancer. That's one powerful habit!

Serving Size Deception

Research shows that people underestimate their caloric intake by around 30%. So this week I want to warn you about foods that **seem** guilt-free, but their calories add up fast if you don't watch the serving size. I see lots of folks gain weight on these seemingly harmless foods:

1) Fat-free whipped cream or Cool Whip: sure it's only 15 calories per serving, but a serving is only 1-2 Tbsp! Almost everything is low-calorie at that portion size! See how much you **really** use and do the math.

2) Fat Free Parmesan Cheese: a serving is 15 calories, but that is for only 2 tsp.

3) Spray Butter: Even though it says 0 calories per serving, it actually is caloric and the manufacturer is rounding down. The second ingredient is oil, so it **is** possible to overdo it if you go nuts with spraying or—I know people do this—take off the top and pour. There are about 900 servings in the container,

so if you finish a container a week, you know you're using enough oil to add up!

4) Low-calorie salad dressing: Same as above—it's only low calorie in small portions. If you like lots of dressing on your salad, consider using gourmet vinegar or salsa.

Have a good week of measuring serving-sizes. It will pay off.

Every Meal Counts!

I have a true tale that shows just how fast your health can change after a few good or bad meals!

Today I met a client who was worried about his cholesterol because it had skyrocketed up to 320, despite his normally healthy diet. His doctor wanted to start him on medication that he would need to take for life.

We went over his diet and couldn't find any problems for cholesterol. Upon further digging, we figured out that for a week preceding his last cholesterol test he had been on vacation eating fried foods, alcohol and very few fruits and veggies. He and his doctor had assumed that one week of abnormal eating couldn't greatly influence a cholesterol test.

...but it can!

He went home and took another test and found his cholesterol was down to 190, a much better number.

This demonstrates how even just a few meals can drastically change your health! Cholesterol, blood sugar and triglycerides can all change radically after just a few bad meals. Newer research is suggesting that just a few healthy meals can immediately improve your resistance to cancer, and I wouldn't be surprised if your immune system, mood and all kinds of other health indices change fast too. Every meal counts!

The Corporate Athlete

Just like serious athletes use sports nutrition to stay strong and fast, the "corporate athletes"—those people who demand high achievement at work all week—need to use nutrition as a performance tool.

Nutrition can make all the difference to corporate performance because it affects mood, memory, mental stamina and cognitive endurance—all the things an executive or office worker uses to be their best.

The highest priority for the corporate athlete is to have optimal blood sugar throughout the day. The brain runs on blood sugar and can't access energy from fat the way muscles can. This means that low blood sugar will make mood, memory and thinking slow down and suffer.

The solution is frequent low-glycemic snacks. Think fruit, string cheese, nuts, seeds, low-sugar yogurt, cottage cheese, sandwiches, salads, soups, and most foods that are unprocessed. By eating these snacks every few hours, the corporate athlete will notice that they think better all day, are less exhausted at night and are more relaxed for their family.

High performance of any kind—mental, cognitive or physical—needs great nutrition.

"Gatorade" for the Corporate Athlete

Yesterday I discussed nutrition for the "Corporate Athlete" and touted frequent low-glycemic snacks as the key to great performance. Whereas solid food snacks are the best option, many Corporate Athletes are too busy to stop and eat every few hours during long meetings, while traveling or while interacting with clients. Here's the solution:

A mug full of almond milk, soymilk, lowfat milk or Imagine brand soup.

Imagine soups are available at Trader Joe's or health food stores and come in a variety of flavors, such as tomato, creamy broccoli, portabella mushroom and butternut squash. They are creamy from soymilk, not cream, so they have a bit of protein without the saturated fat.

Why are they "Gatorade" for the Corporate Athlete?

You can slowly sip on them throughout the day and they will keep your blood sugar at a nice level. They are low in calories, low-glycemic and nobody knows you are drinking soup instead of coffee. You can prepare the soup in seconds by either microwaving it in a mug or just mixing it with hot water.

Try it and see how much better you feel. Not only will your mood and memory be better throughout the day, but come nighttime you won't be as ravenously hungry. They are a great performance food that should always be available in your desk drawer.

Taming the Dog Brain

I believe we shouldn't feel so guilty for eating poorly on occasion. It's in our nature to do so and my dog, Jasper, reminds me of that every day. He will eat almost anything he sees—garbage, dirty socks, tissues—and will beg for more dog food whenever he isn't busy doing something else.

Jasper reminds us that animals are biologically designed to eat whenever possible. Evolutionarily this makes sense, since food scarcity was the biggest danger until the last few hundred years.

Humans have big powerful brains that give us willpower, good judgment and self-control, and we don't give ourselves enough credit for using these skills to overcome the dog brain underneath. Unfortunately our big brains also give us *guilt* when the primitive dog brain underneath succeeds in making us overeat.

Give yourself a break...or maybe a leash? Your choice.

Food Pushers

We all know "food pushers", those well-intentioned (or not) family or friends who are intent on getting us to "just have a bite." They make us eat to avoid feeling rude or embarrassed, but unfortunately food eaten *for* them still ends up in *our* fat cells!

Defend yourself by preparing some phrases or strategies you can use next time. Practice them so you'll be ready. Here are some examples:

- "I'm just too full right now, but I'd love to take some for later."

- "I can't eat another bite, but it was delicious! Can I have the recipe?"

- "I just brushed my teeth, so I'll wait a few hours."

- "I know my husband would *love* this. Let me package this up and take some to him."

A few planned phrases go a long way in this "food means love" culture of ours, so take a minute right now to think of some you can use.

Variety is Overrated

It turns out that being in a food rut can actually help you lose weight! Who knew!?

Even though dietary variety is good for nutrition, it makes you eat more. Studies show that when people eat the same foods often, they eat less **without even knowing it!** Use this to your advantage by doing some of the following:

- Cook a big pot of something healthy once a week and eat it for several meals.

- Plan to have the same super-healthy meal every Monday night to get your week off to a good start.

- Put a few healthy foods on your "permanent grocery list" so that you always have them around (e.g. apples, chicken breasts, frozen stir-fry veggies and Ready-Pac salad greens).

These things also make cooking a lot simpler, so now you can use your extra time and creativity to spice up your workouts!

Finally, an excuse to be boring!

Burn Fat Faster

You probably already know that unsaturated fats (olive oil, nuts, avocado, fatty fish) are a lot healthier for your heart than saturated fats (butter, cream, beef), but get this: new research suggests that our ***bodies burn UNsaturated fat more easily than other fats***. That means it is easier to lose weight if the fat came from those healthier sources. So here are some ways to replace saturated fats with unsaturated ones:

- Use olive or canola oils instead of butter.

- Eat more fish and less beef.

- Use nonfat dairy products.

- Replace cheese with nuts, nut butter, or seeds.

- Avoid salad dressing unless it is nonfat or you know it was made with olive or canola oil.

This is not a free pass to eat good fats! They are just as caloric as the bad ones and can still make you gain weight, so don't increase your overall fat intake, just replace the bad fats with the good.

Remember Your Meals

As the holiday junk food gets more plentiful and your willpower wanes, here's a simple strategy for preventing overeating: *think about your last meal.*

A recent study revealed that people ate less at a meal when they were first prompted to remember what they had eaten at their last one. So as you set the table or make your way to a restaurant, make a mental note of the foods you ate at your last sitting. Simple, eh?

Holiday Health

Today I want you to get your creative juices flowing to think about how you can make your next birthday, anniversary, holiday or other special occasion *not revolve around food!*

Hopefully you are going to have lots of special occasions in your lifetime, so you can't afford to indulge at every one. So here are some ideas for things you could do instead of just going out for a big meal.

Birthday ideas:

- Have a mini-golf tournament.
- Get a group together for a yoga class to prove you're not old.
- Do something silly, like go country line dancing,

Anniversary ideas:

- Go out dancing or take a dance lesson.
- Go for a walk on the beach.
- Hike to a beautiful place.
- Go for a scenic drive.

Holidays with kids:

- Go hiking with your family on Easter to celebrate Springtime.
- Play a game in the park with your family.
- Go bowling.
- Do arts and crafts.
- Play a board game.
- Have a picnic.
- Create a treasure hunt or scavenger hunt.

Other celebrations:

- Have a spa day.
- Get massages.
- Go to a theme park (and bring your own healthy snacks).
- Go to a climbing wall, batting cage, etc.
- Ride horses.
- Play video games at an arcade.

These things might take some extra effort, but they're more fun than just pigging out and you won't have the day-after guilt trip!

Breathe Deep

Take a moment right now to take a slow deep breath. Feel the air go all the way down to your abdomen. Many people go for hours shallow breathing (where only your chest fills with air, not your entire abdomen.) This can lead to muscle tension, headaches, poor posture and a lack of oxygen. Taking a deep breath more often can help relieve stress, give you more energy, improve concentration and increase your metabolism.

Easy, eh?

Nice Legs

Not always motivated to eat fruits and veggies for your health? Then how about for *nice legs*?!

Eating more fruits and veggies can prevent varicose veins. Studies show that the flavenoids found in fruits and veggies such as cherries, blueberries, broccoli and carrots may improve chronic venous insufficiency, a condition that can lead to varicose veins. Apparently, flavenoids can improve the elasticity and tone of veins to keep them—and your legs—looking and feeling young.

A Sweet Treat You Should Eat

Did you know that eating more fruit in the morning helps prevent craving sweets in the afternoon and evening? Try it—it works! And don't miss berry season. The fountain of youth (or the closest thing to it) is in those delicious berries!

Plan, Man

I've noticed over the years that the healthiest eaters aren't the ones with the best knowledge, motivation or intentions, but the ones with the best *preparation*.

An eating plan makes all the difference in our busy lives. In fact, the healthiest eaters are often the people who make a food plan in advance and then are too busy *not* to stick to it!

Try this and I bet you'll eat healthier and lose weight the next few days: write down exactly what you plan to eat for meals and snacks the next 3 days. Think about where you'll be for meals and whether you need to bring something with you. Now plan *when* you will get to the store and prepare these foods. Schedule this time in your calendar and make it sacred, like an important appointment. Do this *now* and see what a difference a plan makes!

Blossoming (Taste) Buds

Did you know that your taste buds grow more sensitive to subtle flavors when you cut back on salt, sugar and fat? It takes a couple of weeks, but if you stop eating over-flavored foods you will start to notice that previously bland foods taste wonderful.

For example, brown rice (sans soy sauce) and air-popped popcorn (no butter or salt) will start to have a nutty flavor. Carrots, peas and corn will taste deliciously sweet, and a baked yam will be guilt-free heaven! Believe it or not, you will start to prefer your foods au natural because their flavors are more complex and interesting than the tastes of added salt, sugar and fat.

Of course, healthier foods will taste bland until your taste buds adjust, but it's worth it! Invest two weeks to start really enjoying healthy flavors again.

Mush Burgers

Have you tried portabella mushrooms lately? They're delicious, meaty, filling and only 20 calories for a mushroom the size of a large hamburger! I put them on my list of greatest foods because they are so easy, convenient, healthy and low-calorie. You can eat them like a burger, on skewers with other veggies, stir fried or however you like. They cook best with a coating of balsamic vinegar and a light spray of canola oil. You can grill them, broil them or even put them on your George Foreman Grill. You are all better cooks than I am, so let me know what other recipes you come up with!

Got Crab?

If you are getting bored of eating chicken and fish all the time, then consider fresh crab. As long as you skip the butter sauce, it's the perfect nutritious, low-calorie, fat-free protein and it's fun to eat. If you get the whole crab and dig out the meat yourself, your meal will also serve as your entertainment and keep you from eating too fast. If you don't mind getting a little messy, it's the perfect fun and interactive meal.

Sit Up and...

Are you slouching right now? Well, stop it!

Sitting up nice and straight will not only make you **look** ten pounds thinner, but will also burn extra calories by engaging your abdominal and back muscles. Think of sitting up straighter every time you hear a phone ring or stop at a red light. These constant reminders will help you turn good posture into a habit so that you'll have it all day long.

...and if I don't already sound enough like your mother, "Eat your vegetables!"

Plan to be Lazy

Do you ever get home for the evening and feel too tired to cook? Ever forget to plan ahead and have to come up with a meal at the last minute? *Of course you do!* Domino's pizza and McDonalds count on it. These situations won't ruin your diet if you keep some of these healthy, easy, "emergency" foods in your house at all times:

KEEP THESE IN THE FREEZER:

- frozen veggies (to steam, stir-fry, make omelets, or add to canned soups)
- Skillet Sensations or other similar frozen stir-fry
- frozen chicken breasts, turkey, or fish filets
- veggie burgers
- Egg Beaters (to make omelets with veggies)
- frozen ostrich burgers (as tasty as beef, but much healthier)
- frozen fruit (to add to yogurt, oatmeal)
- healthy frozen ravioli (e.g. Whole Foods has some filled with veggies or chicken instead of

cheese and you can add more of your own frozen veggies to the sauce)

NON-PERISHABLES FOR THE CUPBOARD:

- water-packed tuna or salmon
- rolled oats
- Fantastic Foods Chili Mix + canned beans + canned tomatoes
- low-fat, low-sodium Raman noodles (add extra water and your own frozen veggies)
- low-sodium broth-based soups (Healthy Valley and Pritikin are two good choices)
- low-sodium broth (throw in your own protein and veggies)
- popcorn kernels (for air-popping)

TRY TO ALWAYS KEEP THESE IN YOUR FRIDGE:

- non-fat cottage cheese (try the low-sodium kind)
- non-fat yogurt
- bagged lettuce
- baby carrots or sugar snap peas
- low-fat string cheese
- hardboiled eggs

Having a stash of healthy "emergency foods" makes **all the difference** when you are busy or tired, so keep this list handy. Print it out and take it with you grocery shopping.

That's All for Now

These are my favorite tips from the last few years, and more are coming out all the time. I'll be sure to keep blogging about them at http://jillsblog.dietforhealth.com, and I'd love to hear what works for you personally. We can never have enough healthy ideas, tricks, strategies or victories, so please share yours. I'm at jill@dietforhealth.com, and I always love hearing from you!

-Jill

About the Author

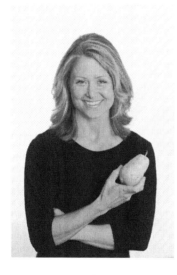

Jill Brook, M.A. is the owner of Diet for Health, an award-winning nutrition practice in Southern California dedicated to helping people find their own most painless ways to look, feel and *be* their very best.

Jill received her degrees from Princeton University and UCLA and then worked as a nutrition and weight loss researcher at UCLA and the Pritikin Longevity Center, studying why *knowing* how to eat right doesn't help people *do* it. Jill now spends her time helping her clients work smarter at achieving their weight and fitness goals. She also writes books, leads workshops, consults for universities and food companies and occasionally appears on television. Visit her at www.dietforhealth.com.

11623441R0013

Made in the USA
Lexington, KY
18 October 2011